The Microbiological Safety of Food

Part II

Report of the Committee on the Microbiological Safety of Food to the Secretary of State for Health, the Minister of Agriculture, Fisheries and Food, and the Secretaries of State for Wales, Scotland and Northern Ireland

Chairman: Sir Mark Richmond

London: HMSO

ISBN 0 11 321347 6

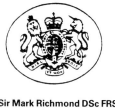

Sir Mark Richmond DSc FRS
Chairman

SCIENCE AND ENGINEERING RESEARCH COUNCIL

Polaris House
North Star Avenue
Swindon
SN2 1ET

Telephone (switchboard) 0793 411000
Direct Line 0793 411291
Fax 0793 411099
Telex 449466

Our Ref: HSt.F.01

21 November 1990

Dear Secretary of State,

    I am now sending you a copy of the second and final part of our Report "The Microbiological Safety of Food".

    My colleagues and I would be pleased to discuss the contents of the Report with you if you would find it helpful.

Yours sincerely

Mark Richmond

The Rt. Hon. William Waldegrave M.P.,
Secretary of State for Health,
Department of Health,
Richmond House,
79 Whitehall,
London,
SW1A 2NS

The Rt. Hon. John Gummer, M.P.,
Minister of Agriculture, Fisheries and Food,
Whitehall Place,
London,
SW1A 2HH

The Rt. Hon. Malcolm Rifkind, Q.C., M.P.,
Secretary of State for Scotland,
Dover House,
Whitehall,
London,
SW1A 2AU

The Rt. Hon. David Hunt, M.B.E., M.P.,
Secretary of State for Wales,
Gwydyr House,
Whitehall,
London,
SW1A 2ER

The Rt. Hon Peter Brooke, M.P.,
Secretary of State for Northern Ireland,
Whitehall,
London,
SW1A 2AZ

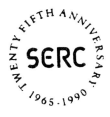

(i)

(ii)

LIST OF MEMBERS

CHAIRMAN
Professor Sir Mark Richmond PhD, ScD, FRCPath, FRS
Vice Chancellor, University of Manchester

MEMBERS
Professor J P Arbuthnott BSc, PhD, ScD, F Inst Biol
Professor of Microbiology, University of Nottingham

Dr A C Baird-Parker OBE, BSc, PhD
Head of Microbiology, Unilever Research Laboratories

Mr D Clarke MIBiol
Food Technology Manager, Trusthouse Forte

Mr B P Denyer DMS, MIEH, FBIM
Director of Environmental Services, City of Westminster

Dr N S Galbraith CBE, FRCP, FFCM
Epidemiologist, Former Director, Communicable Disease Surveillance Centre

Professor G Glew BSc, MSc, C Biol, MIFST, FHCIMA
Emeritus Professor, Hotel and Catering Research Centre, Huddersfield
Polytechnic

Mr A M Johnston BVM&S, MRCVS, FRSH
Senior Lecturer, Royal Veterinary College, University of London

Mr J E Moffitt CBE, DCL, FRASE
Farmer

Professor J R Norris, BSc, PhD, DSc, F Inst Biol
Director of Group Research, Cadbury-Schweppes Plc

Dr R Spencer MSc, PhD, FIFST, F Inst Biol
Director of Scientific Services, J Sainsbury Plc

Dame Rachel Waterhouse, PhD
Chairman, Consumers Association

ASSESSORS
Miss R D B Pease
Department of Health

Mr B H B Dickinson
Ministry of Agriculture, Fisheries and Food

SECRETARIAT
Dr R Skinner MD MSc MRCPath
Medical Secretary
Department of Health

Miss M L Ferguson
Department of Health

Mr C J Ryder
Administrative Secretary
Ministry of Agriculture, Fisheries and Food

Mr J O'Gorman
Ministry of Agriculture, Fisheries and Food

CONTENTS

FIGURES

TABLES

CHAPTER 1

INTRODUCTION

1.1 The Secretary of State for Health, on behalf of the UK Health and Agriculture Ministers, announced in the House of Commons on 21 February 1989 (Hansard Column 877) the setting up of a Committee on the Microbiological Safety of Food, to be chaired by Sir Mark Richmond, Professor of Molecular Microbiology and Vice-Chancellor, University of Manchester. The Committee was given the following terms of reference:—

> "To advise the Secretary of State for Health, the Minister of Agriculture, Fisheries and Food and the Secretaries of State for Wales, Scotland and Northern Ireland, on matters remitted to it by Ministers relating to the microbiological safety of food and on such matters as it considers need investigation."

1.2 Ministers asked the Committee to look at specific questions relating to the increasing incidence of microbiological illnesses of foodborne origin, particularly from salmonella, listeria and campylobacter; to establish whether this is linked to changes in agriculture and food production, food technology and distribution, retailing, catering and food handling in the home and to recommend action where appropriate.

1.3 Subsequently the Secretary of State for Health asked the Committee to consider the implications of the outbreak of botulism in June 1989 caused by the use of inadequately processed hazelnut puree in the manufacture of yoghurt.

1.4 The Committee consisted of eleven members in addition to the Chairman. The membership was announced by the Secretary of State for Health on 23 March 1989. An assessor from the Department of Health (DH) and from the Ministry of Agriculture, Fisheries and Food (MAFF) attended each meeting to help provide information for the Committee. The Secretariat was provided jointly by DH and MAFF.

1.5 It is with deep regret that we report the death of one of our members, Professor George Glew, on 12 August 1990. Professor Glew made a major contribution to the Committee's work, particularly on catering matters.

THE COMMITTEE'S FIRST REPORT

1.6 The Committee's first report to the Ministers — *The Microbiological Safety of Food: Part I* — was published on 15 February 1990. At the same time the Government published its response to the Committee's recommendations. The recommendations and the response are reproduced as Appendix 1 to this part of our report.

1.7 For ease of reference and for greater continuity between the two parts of our report, we reproduce below the summary of the contents of Part I:—

"*Chapter 2* briefly examines the epidemiological data (including those of the Public Health Laboratory Service (PHLS) and of the Office of Population Censuses and

Surveys (OPCS) on foodborne illness in humans, and those of the Veterinary Investigation Service (VIS) of MAFF's State Veterinary Service on zoonoses), so as to establish the trends in the incidence of the principal microorganisms of concern. A more comprehensive examination of the epidemiological data on salmonella, campylobacter and listeria is at Appendices 1, 2, & 3.

"*Chapter 3* then examines in detail the PHLS and VIS systems for epidemiological surveillance, and in particular the arrangements for central collation and review of the data, for liaison between the veterinary and medical sides, for identifying actual or potential health problems, and for instituting action both at central and local government level. We make a number of recommendations in these areas. We also conclude that it is important to establish more precisely the extent of gastrointestinal disease in the population.

"*Chapter 4* examines the arrangements for handling outbreaks of foodborne illness, and in particular the roles of the various bodies and organisations which are involved centrally and locally. We make recommendations for improved liaison and co-ordination.

"*Chapter 5* considers the way food is surveyed at present. The present arrangements for the microbiological surveillance of food are largely ad hoc. We recommend that a formalised committee structure be set up to coordinate such food surveillance in the future, and to consider the results in the context of all other available data; this should enable the establishment of a formal structure to ensure a co-ordinated development of food safety policy.

"*Chapter 6* covers the production of raw poultry meat up to the end of the slaughter process.

"*Chapter 7* deals with the manufacturing process, particularly as applied to meat and dairy products.

"*Chapter 8* reports on the results of a limited study which we conducted into food processing by smaller enterprises, in view of the increasing popularity of "natural" or home-made foods from such sources.

"*Chapter 9* deals with legislative matters. We have already commented to Ministers on some of these. The subjects covered are:—

a. content of the Food Safety Bill;

b. the Government's proposed revision of the Food Hygiene Regulations;

c. the Government's proposals relating to the sale of unpasteurised cows' milk;

d. the Report "Public Health in England";

e. review of law on infectious disease control;

f. food labelling requirements in relation to shelf life;

g. performance criteria for refrigerators.

"*Chapter 10* draws together and summarises the main conclusions and recommendations reached in the first part of our report."

1.8 We completed work in Committee for this second and final part of our report — as Ministers had asked — by 31 July 1990, although postal consultation continued until October 1990. Part II contains the following further chapters:—

Chapter 1 introduces Part II, and surveys events and developments that have occurred since the publication of Part I.

Chapter 2 draws out the most important general themes and conclusions that have emerged from the Committee's work.

Chapter 3 examines the arrangements in Scotland and Northern Ireland for gathering and collating epidemiological data and identifying problems on both the human and veterinary sides; for managing outbreaks; and for food surveillance.

Chapters 4, 5 and 6 cover production of the foodstuffs outstanding after Part I which are of most relevance from a microbiological safety of food point of view, and which it is practical to examine at this time — red meat, milk and milk products, fish and shellfish.

Chapters 7, 8, 9 and 10 deal with the later stages of the food chain — the transport of food, retailing and wholesaling, catering, and the consumer and the home.

Chapter 11 draws together and develops our conclusions, from both parts of our report, about education and training.

Chapter 12 summarises and develops the views on research from both parts of the report.

Chapter 13 summarises the recommendations from this part of our report (those from Part I being set out at Appendix 1, as noted above).

Three further Appendices set out epidemiological information as follows:—

Appendix 2 on Botulism

Appendix 3 on Viral Foodborne Disease

Appendix 4 on Other Relevant Pathogens.

1.9 The Committee met eleven times since publication of Part I of our report, including a weekend meeting. As was the case previously, preparatory work for particular parts of our report was undertaken by small groups of Committee members, and therefore involved a considerable number of additional meetings.

**THE SCOPE OF THE
COMMITTEE'S WORK**

1.10 The Committee was set up at a time when there was particular concern about salmonella in eggs. As we noted in Part I, paragraph 1.11(e), the subject has been covered in depth by the House of Commons Select Committee on Agriculture (in a report presented to Parliament in February 1989 and in a subsequent progress report in December 1989).

1.11 We noted in Part I, paragraphs 6.12 — 6.14, that the Government had introduced a wide ranging package of measures (whose up-to-date chronology is set out at Annex 1.1 to this chapter), and we stated that the measures represented as comprehensive an approach to the salmonella problem as had — so far as we were aware — been adopted anywhere in the world. This conclusion still holds. In Part I we stressed the importance of assessing their effects in a coordinated way, and we therefore decided to defer our own consideration of eggs.

1.12 However, even now, many of the measures designed to control the situation have been in operation for less than a year, as Annex 1.1 shows. We therefore feel it is <u>still</u> too early to draw firm conclusions.

1.13 We have already recommended (Part I, paragraph 5.32) the establishment of a Steering Group and Advisory Committee structure to provide a national microbiological surveillance and assessment system. The Secretary of State for Health subsequently announced to the House of Commons the Government's intention of setting up such a structure (see paragraph 1.21(b) below). We therefore **recommend that the topic of eggs should be considered by the Steering Group and Advisory Committee on the Microbiological Safety of Food as soon as possible in their programmes of work** (R(II)1.1).

1.14 The topic of waterborne illness of microbial origin is outside our terms of reference, and illness due to Cryptosporidium in particular is the subject of a recent report to Ministers, "Cryptosporidium in Water Supplies", by a Committee under the Chairmanship of Sir John Badenoch. This was published on 20 July 1990.

1.15 Similarly, we have not addressed Bovine Spongiform Encephalopathy (BSE). A Committee chaired by Dr David Tyrrell is advising the Government on this subject.

RECENT AND FORTHCOMING DEVELOPMENTS

1.16 The following paragraphs review developments which have occurred since publication of Part I — and some which can be foreseen — under the following headings:—

— latest information on foodborne illness;

— Government action;

— Institution of Environmental Health Officers/Audit Commission survey of food premises;

— action by industry;

— future statutory requirements: the EC dimension;

— the licensing issue.

Latest information on foodborne illness

1.17 Since publication of Part I of our report in February 1990, 1989 figures have become available in the various data series for England and Wales and can be found in Chapter 3 below, at Tables 3.2, 3.3 and 3.4. In addition to the weekly statistics available in the Communicable Disease Report (CDR) (see Part I, paragraph 3.12), the PHLS — SVS have published further editions of their quarterly 'Update on Salmonella Infection'. Also, the PHLS Communicable Disease Surveillance Centre (CDSC) published a report in April analysing the 1,562 outbreaks reported to CDSC over the three-year period 1986-1988, a helpful analysis which is referred to at a number of points in this report.

1.18 Since we finalised Part I, the main trends to emerge in England and Wales from data published on statutory notifications of food poisoning and from returns relating to particular pathogens are as follows:—

Notifications of food poisoning. The number of cases, formally notified and "ascertained by other means", reported to the Office of Population Censuses and Surveys (OPCS) during 1989 continued the upward trend of previous years. The total was 52,492 compared with 39,713 in 1988, an increase of 32% (data for 1975-1989 are shown in Table 3.1 in Part II, Chapter 3). However, in the first three quarters of 1990 there was a small decrease of 5.8% compared with the same period of 1989. These data may be particularly influenced by variations in the proportions of cases notified.

Salmonellosis. The number of isolates of all salmonellas from humans in England and Wales sent to the PHLS Division of Enteric Pathogens (DEP) in 1989 was 29,998, compared with 27,478 for 1988, a 9% increase. Within this total S.enteritidis PT4 increased by 3%. The total number decreased by 6.8% in the first 9 months of 1990 to 20,350 from 21,843 in the same period of 1989 (see Part I, paragraph 2.10), but within this total S.enteritidis PT4 increased by 15% with corresponding reductions in other serotypes.

In addition to these DEP data, a separate but not directly comparable set of data derived from reports of laboratory isolations sent to CDSC is published in the CDR. Laboratory reports to CDSC of total salmonellas in England and Wales for 1989 were 24,732 compared with 23,821 for 1988, an increase of 3.8%. Within this total S.enteritidis PT4 increased by 5.6%. As in the DEP data, there was a similar fall of total reports in 1990; in the first 39 weeks of the year this was 6.4%, from 17,413 in 1989 to 16,298. There was also a similar but smaller proportionate increase in reports of S.enteritidis PT4 over this period from 6,889 in 1989 to 7,678 in 1990 (11.5%). **We reiterate most strongly our recommendation (Part I, paragraph 3.46) that the PHLS should take steps to eliminate the confusion that can potentially arise from the lack of comparability between the two data sets (R(II)1.2).**

Campylobacter enteritis. There were 32,526 laboratory reports to the CDSC of Campylobacter infection in England and Wales in 1989 compared with 28,761 reports in 1988, an increase of 13.1%. In the first 39 weeks of 1990 there was a smaller increase of 3.3% (from 25,814 to 26,607) compared with the same period in 1989.

Listeriosis. The total number of cases of listeriosis reported to CDSC in 1989 was 250 compared with 291 in 1988, a decrease of 14%. In the first nine months of 1990 only 90 cases of listeriosis were reported to CDSC, a fall of 61% from the figure of 228 for the comparable period of 1989. Reports from Scotland and from Northern Ireland in the first nine months of 1990 were also reduced compared with previous years. We believe that this decline in the reported incidence of listeriosis in the United Kingdom reflects a significant change. In Part I, Appendix 3, we referred to the fact that some samples of soft cheeses and pate were found to contain large numbers of organisms, particularly serotype 4 which was the most frequently isolated from man. The downturn in the reported incidence of listeriosis may be related to increased awareness among the public, and among all others involved in the food chain, of the risks and of the precautions to be taken.

1.19 Information on statutory notifications and returns relating to particular pathogens in Scotland and in Northern Ireland is discussed in Part II, Chapter 3. In our consideration of the problem of foodborne disease we found that there were differences in the way information was collected, collated and reported between the constituent countries of the UK such that reported statistics were not directly comparable. We comment on this in several places in Chapter 3 below. **We recommend that the Steering Group on the Microbiological Safety of Food should consult all the countries of the UK with a view to putting data collection and reporting on a commonly agreed basis** (R(II)1.3).

Government action

1.20 Since we completed Part I, the most important development in the field of food safety in the United Kingdom has been the passage into law of the Food Safety Act 1990. The Act sets a framework within which many of our recommendations can be implemented, providing new and stronger powers to protect the public against food hazards. In addition, in July 1990 the Government laid regulations before Parliament amending and extending the temperature control requirements of the Food Hygiene Regulations. The need for tighter control of temperature is a recurring theme in our report, and we therefore welcome this.

1.21 In relation to the recommendations in Part I of our report we are pleased to note the following developments:—

(a) the setting up by DH of two pilot studies to be run concurrently — the first to investigate the incidence of infectious intestinal disease in the community, and the second to investigate cases of infectious gastrointestinal disease seen by general practitioners. The studies have been designed, and are being co-ordinated, by the Communicable Disease Surveillance Centre (CDSC) and DH with the assistance of the PHLS microbiologists, the Epidemiology and Medical Care Unit of the Medical Research Council (MRC), and the London School of Hygiene and Tropical Medicine. If these studies are satisfactory, we expect that a full-scale national survey will be undertaken, which would address the recommendation in Part I, paragraphs 3.35 and 3.36. Such a national survey should lead to important improvements in the information available on the incidence of infectious gastrointestinal disease where the diagnosis has been confirmed by microbiological examination;

(b) the announcement (reproduced at Annex 1.2), of the Government's intention to establish (i) a Steering Group and (ii) an Advisory Committee on the Microbiological Safety of Food. This extremely important decision meets our key recommendation (see Part I, paragraph 5.22) for a national microbiological surveillance and assessment system. We understand that membership will be drawn from all parts of the UK, and we are confident that these new arrangements can provide a sound basis for future policy decisions and action in relation to the microbiological safety of food;

(c) the strengthening of the statutory measures in relation to poultry and egg production (described in Part I, paragraph 6.12) in the following ways:—

— the slaughter policy for poultry flocks in which *S.enteritidis* or *S.typhimurium* is confirmed — which originally applied to laying flocks only — has been progressively extended to layer-breeder and broiler-breeder flocks;

— the registration of laying flocks of over 100 birds, and of breeding flocks and hatcheries as defined, has been required from 2 April 1990;

— on 11 June 1990 a consultation document was circulated in connection with draft Egg Products Regulations which would set higher standards for the manufacture of egg products;

— the ban on the sale of cracked eggs from packing stations was extended to cover sales direct from producer to consumer (eg farm gate sales) from 31 July 1990;

(d) the various initiatives which have been taken to improve the flow of information to the public on the microbiological safety of food. Among these are the monthly Food Safety Information Bulletin from MAFF's Food Safety Directorate (which includes input from both the Agriculture and Health Departments), and school packs and videos aimed at improving food hygiene awareness among school children and the general public. Also, MAFF's Consumer Panel has had its first meetings, and papers presented to it, together with the record of its discussions, are made freely available to the public and to the press;

(e) the Government's proposal that "sell by" dates will no longer be permitted, that "use by" dates will be introduced for highly perishable foods with effect from 1 January 1991, and that it will be an offence to sell food after its "use by" date. This will meet our recommendation in Part I, paragraph 9.25;

(f) the work that is now going on with the assistance of the Implementation Advisory Committee to prepare statutory codes of practice for issue by Ministers under section 40 of the Food Safety Act 1990 to guide enforcement authorities towards an even and consistent standard of enforcement. We highlighted this need in Part I, Annex 9.1;

(g) the guidelines which have been circulated for public comment on compliance with the Food Hygiene (Amendment) Regulations 1990 (mentioned at paragraph 1.20 above);

(h) Department of Health's consultation on the training of food handlers, on the basis of proposals they issued on 5 December 1989. We have highlighted the importance of education and training throughout both parts of our report, and a resumé of our views, together with a copy of our response to DH's consultation document, is at Part II, Chapter 11;

(i) the report published in September 1990 by the Welsh Office reviewing the local arrangements for the handling of a food poisoning outbreak affecting some 640 people (3 deaths) which occurred in Clwyd, North Wales and Cheshire during July/August 1989. The outbreak was caused by inadequately cooked meat contaminated by *S.typhimurium* DT12. The report drew attention to the need for those involved in management of outbreaks, particularly the Local Authority and Proper Officer, to be fully resourced and aware of their responsiblities, and for all relevant information to be passed to the appropriate officials as soon as possible. We believe the report's conclusions reinforce our recommendation at Part I, paragraph 4.44, that responsibilities for the management of outbreaks be clarified. The report also reinforces our concerns (see Part I, paragraphs 4.11 and 4.12) about the difficulties of developing an integrated response to outbreaks which span a number of authority boundaries. The Welsh Office has now issued a health circular setting out advice on producing guidance on the handling of serious outbreaks of food poisoning and has asked District Councils to draw up plans in liaison with District Health Authorities for dealing with such outbreaks. As noted in Part II, Chapter 3, guidance on this topic is being drafted in Scotland, and has been issued in Northern Ireland. This highlights the importance of a consistency of approach to the management of outbreaks in the constituent countries of the UK (see Part II, paragraph 3.24).

Institution of Environmental Health Officers/Audit Commission Survey of Food Premises

1.22 In preparing this second part of our report we have had the benefit of seeing the results of a national Food Premises Condition Survey, organised by the Audit Commission for Local Authorities in England and Wales in co-operation with the Institution of Environmental Health Officers (IEHO) (Audit Commission Report No 2, June 1990). The survey covered over 5,000 premises inspected by environmental health officers (EHOs) in England and Wales. The survey data, which the Audit Commission has kindly allowed us to analyse further, help to show where, in the professional judgement of EHOs, food safety is put at risk, the reasons for this and the severity of the risk. The survey has provided a useful complement to reports on outbreaks of foodborne disease and the food poisoning statistics provided by the OPCS and the PHLS.

1.23 Overall, the survey suggests that, in the judgement of EHOs, almost one in eight food premises in England and Wales presents a significant or imminent health risk. Of these, they considered that one third should be prosecuted or closed down. Take-aways, and some food manufacturers and restaurants, cafés and canteens were found to present the most risk (the sample of food manufacturers did not typify the food manufacturing sector because it was weighted towards smaller businesses); hospitals, residential homes and educational establishments the least risk. Large metropolitan areas have significantly more high-risk premises than the rest of the country. The factors most commonly assessed as leading to high risks were ineffective monitoring of temperatures, poor staff hygiene awareness, the risk of cross-contamination arising from poor practices, inadequate hand washing facilities and a lack of hygiene awareness on the part of management. In addition most high-risk premises were in poor physical condition. A summary of our additional analyses is at Annex 1.3, and in our view reinforces many of our recommendations, including those for licensing.

Action by Industry

1.24 The food industry, too, has been active in ensuring that the highest standards of food safety are achieved and maintained. We understand that individual businesses have improved their practices and processes in relation to particular foods identified as being at a high risk from microbiological contamination. Also, various trade associations have issued further codes of practice covering new and developing technologies. Codes and guidelines outlining good operating practice contribute to the development of awareness of potential risk factors and of the steps which can be taken to minimise those risks. Where appropriate we have drawn attention to specific codes in the individual chapters of both parts of our Report.

Future statutory requirements: the European Community dimension

1.25 The European Community (EC) now has a major role in determining the law on food safety. As part of progress towards establishing the Single European Market by 1993, the EC Commission has produced a range of legislative proposals designed to eliminate non-tariff barriers to trade by ensuring that the same food does not have to meet different requirements in different parts of the Community. The Commission's Agriculture Directorate (DG VI) has proposed a series of draft "vertical" measures (each of which sets requirements for the hygienic production of particular products of animal origin) as well as a measure laying down generalised rules for the handling of such products. DG VI is also preparing important proposals for "horizontal" measures on zoonoses control and on animal waste. The Internal Market Directorate (DG III) has generated a number of food law proposals, which have already been adopted by the Council of Ministers, including ones for:—

— the official control of foodstuffs (which largely concerns inspection arrangements);

— labelling;

— batch-marking.

A Directive on food hygiene — which will lay down general food hygiene rules — is also to be proposed by DG III, and the Commission has informally circulated a preliminary draft for public comment.

1.26 In order to prepare the UK's negotiating position, the Government has circulated for public comment all the proposals which have so far been published by the EC Commission. We have commented, where relevant, on these proposals at various points in our detailed examination of the food chain.

1.27 It is evident — especially given the arrangements for the EC Council of Ministers to adopt measures by qualified majority voting — that many of the recommendations we have made about legislation in our report can only be pursued by negotiating in the Community context. We draw two particular conclusions from this:—

— where the UK already has regulatory controls which it considers important (eg on zoonoses and on food hygiene), the national interest is likely to lie in seeking to ensure that Community measures are adopted on the same lines. Otherwise there is the possibility that the UK's existing stringent controls will be weakened;

— there is also a need to ensure that the two Directorates involved within the Commission adopt a properly coordinated approach. One sign that this is not occurring is that both are contemplating "horizontal" proposals — a regulation on products of animal origin from DG VI, the food hygiene directive from DG III — which would set inconsistent hygiene requirements for the same range of products. This creates unnecessary uncertainty and confusion in the industry over what requirements it may have to meet.

1.28 We understand from MAFF and DH that they attach high priority to addressing these areas in their handling of the EC Commission's proposals. It is clearly of the greatest importance that these problems should be satisfactorily resolved.

The licensing issue

1.29 The Government has taken powers in the Food Safety Act 1990 to provide for the registration and licensing of premises and processes. However, it has made clear (see Part II, Appendix 1) that it does not intend to provide for licensing to the extent we recommended in Part I, paragraph 9.9, but only at present for food irradiation plants, dairy farms and dairies; it intends to propose regulations requiring the registration of all permanent food businesses at least four weeks before opening, and also, where necessary, regulations controlling sensitive processes, such as those involving vacuum packing of food. As explained in Appendix 1, the Government believes that the registration proposals will enable enforcement authorities to direct their enforcement effort to better effect.

1.30 We agree that enforcement officers are in a unique position to provide information and advice to businesses which might otherwise be unaware of the practices they should follow. We therefore **recommend that enforcement officers should take full advantage of registration in order to identify the businesses most in need of attention, and to provide them with information and advice** (R(II))1.4). We refer to this view and other aspects of enforcement in more detail at relevant points in the retailing and catering chapters (Part II, Chapters 8 and 9).

1.31 The actions contemplated by the Government in this area are undoubtedly a step in the right direction (indeed, the registration proposals will meet our recommendation at Part I, paragraph 9.12). However, we greatly regret the Government's decision not to introduce licensing on the scale we recommend and are still of the opinion that licensing of the premises and processes we recommended in Part I ought to be introduced. We have reiterated our recommendations to this effect at Part II, paragraphs 8.49 and 9.59.

ACKNOWLEDGEMENTS 1.32 We should like formally to record here our thanks to the many individuals and organisations who responded to our consultation letter, who submitted papers, talked to the Committee about their particular areas of expertise, or allowed the Committee to visit their factories or institutions as mentioned in the relevant Chapters. A list of those who assisted the Committee in its work is at Annex 1.4.

1.33 We should also like to thank the Secretariat for their support and the Assessors for their advice. However, we stress that we were set up as an independent committee to advise Government and that the views in this report are those of the Committee alone and not necessarily those of the Secretariat, the Assessors, or those providing evidence. To all those who have assisted us we owe a great debt of gratitude.

ANNEX 1.1

SUMMARY OF MAIN LANDMARKS IN THE DEVELOPMENT OF STATUTORY CONTROLS ON SALMONELLA IN EGGS AND POULTRY

1.3.89   Powers taken for compulsory slaughter of poultry, with compensation.

Strengthening of State Veterinary Service (SVS) powers to declare premises infected and impose controls on movements — including the extension of the powers to animal feedingstuffs.

Strengthening of requirements to report positive isolations of salmonella, and extension of requirements to cover isolations from feedingstuffs.

16.3.89   Obligation placed on keepers of laying and breeding flocks to take samples and have them tested for salmonella in accordance with a specified method ("compulsory monitoring").

1.4.89   Ministerial decision to introduce the compulsory slaughter (with compensation) of laying flocks in which *S. enteriditis* or *S. typhimurium* is confirmed.

14.4.89   Processors of animal protein obliged:—

a. to have a sample tested on each day they consign finished product from their premises; and

b. for a period of 28 days, to withhold processed animal protein from incorporation into feedingstuffs if a sample proves positive for salmonella.

1.5.89   New arrangements introduced for inspecting licensed imports of fish or animal protein, so as to concentrate attention on consignments from countries with the poorest record in relation to contamination.

22.5.89   Ministerial decision to extend compulsory slaughter with compensation into layer-breeder sector.

13.6.89   Processors of animal protein obliged to register with MAFF, DAFS or WOAD, as appropriate.

13.8.89   The conduct of statutory tests on processed protein restricted to laboratories authorised by the Minister.

26.10.89   "Compulsory monitoring" requirement (16.3.89 above) extended to hatcheries.

2.11.89   First positive isolation from a layer-breeder flock confirmed, and flock slaughtered.

9.11.89   Ministerial decision to extend compulsory slaughter with compensation to broiler-breeding flocks in which *Salmonella enteriditis* and *Salmonella typhimurium* confirmed.

16.11.89   First broiler-breeder flock slaughtered.

26.3.90	New arrangements concerning slaughter and heat processing announced.
2.4.90	Compulsory registration of poultry flocks introduced.
11.6.90	Consultation document issued, seeking views on draft Egg Products Regulations which would replace the Liquid Egg (Pasteurisation) Regulations 1963 and set higher standards for the manufacture of egg products.
31.7.90	Ban on sale of cracked eggs from packing stations extended to cover sales direct from producer to consumer (eg farm gate sales).

Extent of compulsory slaughter: provisional figures up to week ending 18 November 1990.

No. of Flocks Slaughtered and on which compensation has been paid:

Laying flocks	142
Layer-breeder flocks	4
Broiler-breeder flocks	29
	175

No. of birds slaughtered	1,850,069
Value	£1,829,987

Department of Health

PRESS RELEASE

Richmond House
79 Whitehall
London SW1A 2NS

Telephone 071-210 5963

12 June 1990

ARRANGEMENTS INTRODUCED TO STRENGTHEN FOOD SAFETY MEASURES

Kenneth Clarke, Secretary of State for Health, announced today the establishment of a national microbiological food surveillance and assessment system aimed at improving existing food safety measures.

In a Written Reply to a Parliamentary Question from Simon Burns, MP for Chelmsford, Mr Clarke said: "My Rt hon friend the Minister of Agriculture, Fisheries and Food, and I have decided to establish a national microbiological food surveillance and assessment system. This will be based on a new, independent Advisory Committee on the Microbiological Safety of Food and a new Steering Group on the Microbiological Safety of Food. These arrangements will complement those which already exist for labelling, composition and chemical safety of food, which are within the remit of the present Food Advisory Committee and Steering Group on Food Surveillance.

"The new Steering Group will manage surveillance and research and will present policy conclusions to the Ministers. It will consist both of officials and of experts from outside Government. The Advisory Committee will bring outside expertise to bear on the interpretation of the results of surveillance, and on the policy formation process. The Committee will have an entirely independent membership and chairman, who will be chosen for their expertise and invited from relevant backgrounds, including consumer interests.

"These arrangements will give effect to the recommendation of the present Committee on the Microbiological Safety of Food that the Government should set up a system of microbiological surveillance and assessment. This committee, under the chairmanship of Sir Mark Richmond, has been invited to complete its work by the end of July. The Government plans to establish the new Advisory Committee in the Autumn. The new Steering Group will be established as soon as possible before then, as it can usefully begin preparatory work before the Advisory Committee first meets.

"The membership of the new Advisory Committee and Steering Group, and their formal terms of reference, will be announced as soon as possible. The Food Advisory Committee and the Steering Group on Food Surveillance will continue to fulfil their present functions but some updating of their terms of reference also is envisaged, to underline the complementary roles of this Committee and the new Advisory Committee."

NOTES TO EDITORS

1. The setting up of the Committee on the Microbiological Safety of Food was announced by Kenneth Clarke on 21 February 1989. Its terms of reference are:—

"To advise the Secretary of State for Health, the Minister of Agriculture, Fisheries and Food and the Secretaries of State for Wales, Scotland and Northern Ireland, on matters remitted to it by Ministers relating to the microbiological safety of food and on such matters as it considers need investigation."

The Chairman of the Committee is Sir Mark Richmond, Vice-Chancellor of Manchester University.

2. In the first part of the report "The Microbiological Safety of Food" published on 15 February, the Committee recommended the establishment of a national food and assessment system. In particular, it proposed a structure of two committees: a steering group to coordinate microbiological food safety, and an advisory committee to provide an independent expert view on the public health implications of food safety matters.

3. The Committee has been invited to complete its work by the end of July. The second part of its report is expected to be published in the Autumn.

ANNEX 1.3

ANALYSES OF AUDIT COMMISSION FOOD PREMISES SURVEY DATA

INTRODUCTION

1.3.1 In preparing the second part of our report we have had the benefit of seeing the results of a national Food Premises Condition Survey, organised by the Audit Commission for Local Authorities in England and Wales in co-operation with the Institution of Environmental Health Officers (Audit Commission Report No. 2, June 1990). For further details see Part II, paragraphs 1.22-1.23. This annex details the results of some additional analyses of the source statistics. We concentrated on trying to establish the relationship between health risk and three main factors:—

— physical condition of the premises;

— equipment, practices and hygiene awareness;

— size of premises.

The sample of food manufacturers was weighted towards smaller businesses.

PHYSICAL CONDITION OF PREMISES

1.3.2 Although physical condition of premises does not necessarily cause a health risk, the survey did establish a link between the two: the worse the condition, the higher the health risk (see Exhibit 2 of the Audit Commission Report). We looked at the breakdown of the data to establish how particular aspects of physical condition varied according to types of premises.

1.3.3 In relation to design, structure and condition, ease of cleaning and cleanliness, between 20% and 30% of establishments were generally classed as poor or very poor except for hospitals, educational establishments and residential homes. Food manufacturers generally had the highest proportion of "very poor" cases except with respect to cleanliness where take-aways had the highest proportion, closely followed by restaurants, cafes and canteens. Sanitary conditions seemed to be a problem at take-aways, food manufacturers, other food retailers (eg butchers, fishmongers) and, to a slightly lesser extent, supermarkets, grocers, restaurants, cafes and canteens. Take-aways also had problems with drainage and waste disposal facilities as did food manufacturers, cafes and food retailers.

1.3.4 Hospitals, schools and residential homes consistently outperformed the other types of premises for good physical conditions.

1.3.5 It is clear from the more detailed breakdown of the figures for the retail sector that in general supermarkets rate quite highly, although for cleanliness over 20% were classed as poor or very poor. A quarter or more of grocers were graded as poor or very poor in all respects except drainage and waste disposal facilities. Bakers and butchers showed a broadly similar pattern except that bakers were somewhat better in respect of sanitary conditions and butchers had a slightly superior performance with regard to adequate design and ease of cleaning. Fishmongers appeared to perform quite well generally, but care should be taken in interpreting the results given the small sample (19 premises).

1.3.6 EHOs were asked to make an assessment of health risk arising from 22 different factors. The Audit Commission Report (paragraph 18) listed those factors most commonly assessed as leading to high risks. We looked further at how health risks associated with equipment, practices and hygiene awareness varied among types of premises.

1.3.7 For hotels and guesthouses, the major health risks appeared to stem from poor hand washing facilities, the ineffective monitoring of temperature, the risk of cross-contamination and the lack of hygiene awareness on the part of staff (and, to a lesser degree, of management). There also seemed to be significant problems in restaurants, cafes, canteens, pubs, clubs and bars. However, for restaurants, cafes and canteens there were additional problems of management attitude and the general standard of cleanliness in a large number of premises. With supermarkets, grocers and other food retailers, the incidence of imminent or significant health risks resulting from poor hand washing facilities, poor monitoring of food temperatures, cross-contamination and the lack of hygiene awareness of both staff and management were also high — particularly for "other" food retailers. Another significant problem for food shops seemed to stem from the time/temperature control of foods on display. Besides the low scoring features common to the groups mentioned above, food manufacturers performed relatively poorly with respect to their general standard of cleanliness, the time/temperature control of food in preparation, the application of quality assurance or control systems, hygiene awareness and the use of pest control measures. Take-aways scored badly in a number of respects, but again the main areas of concern appeared to be poor monitoring of temperature, the risk of cross-contamination, the adequacy of hand washing facilities, the lack of hygiene awareness, and management attitude.

1.3.8 The performance of hospitals, educational establishments and residential homes compared very favourably with the other categories. The only major health risk factor identified for these establishments was ineffective monitoring of temperature. Although hygiene awareness was significantly improved over the other categories there was still a large number of premises where this formed a minor risk.

1.3.9 Again we looked more closely at the breakdown of the figures for the retail sector:—

— taking the overall assessment, only just over 6% of supermarkets/ hypermarkets were graded as a significant health risk with none in the imminent category. However, there did seem to be some problems with the time/temperature control of food on display, with monitoring of temperature, with hygiene awareness, and with poor practices and the consequent risk of cross-contamination;

— about one in ten grocers shops was classed as representing a significant health risk, but again there was none in the "imminent risk" category. The main problems identified were inadequate hand washing facilities, ineffective monitoring of temperature, high risks of cross-contamination, and poor hygiene awareness;

— over one in six bakers shops were graded as being an imminent or significant health risk. A large proportion of these shops did not effectively monitor temperature generally, or control the time/temperature of food on display. The lack of hand washing facilities, the degree of hygiene awareness, and the management attitudes towards hygiene were also identified as problems;

— one in eight butchers was in the imminent or significant health risk categories. The risk of cross-contamination from poor practices or equipment was a particular problem; there was also concern over inadequate hand washing facilities, ineffective monitoring of temperature, time/temperature control of food on display and hygiene awareness;

— fishmongers appeared — albeit on the basis of a rather small sample — to compare favourably with other types of shop. They performed well in respect of the monitoring of temperature and time/temperature control of food on display, but inadequate hand washing facilities were noted as a problem.

SIZE OF PREMISES   1.3.10 We also looked at the relationship between establishment size (measured in terms of the number of people handling food) and the overall risk to health. No clear pattern emerged across all types of establishment; for restaurants, supermarkets and grocers, food manufacturers and take-aways the level of risk seemed to diminish as size increased, whereas for hospitals and educational establishments the pattern was reversed. In the case of hotels and guest houses, the best performance was recorded by the smallest establishments and the worst by those with between 20 and 49 people handling food. With pubs, clubs, residential homes and "other" food retailers, there was no discernible relationship between size and risk.

ACKNOWLEDGEMENTS   1.3.11 We are grateful to the Audit Commission who provided the Committee with the detailed statistics collected in their survey and to MAFF's Economics and Statistics (Food) Division for their help in carrying out these additional analyses.

ANNEX 1.4

THOSE WHO HAVE ASSISTED THE COMMITTEE IN ITS WORK

Association of District Councils (Brian Etheridge)

Association of Local Authorities of Northern Ireland (R McKay, Secretary)

Association of Meat Inspectors (Dr J F Gracey, Vice President)

Association of Metropolitan Authorities (Steve Bassam, Assistant Secretary)

Association of Public Analysts (M Barnett, Hon. Secretary)

Audit Commission for Local Authorities in England and Wales

Beverley Borough Council (S R Headley, Principal Environmental Health Officer)

Bolton Health Authority (Dr G N Constable, Director of Public Health)

British Egg Products Association (Colin Parsons, Secretary)

British Goat Society (Ruth Goodwin, Scientific Liaison Officer)

British Poultry Federation (Neville Wallace, Director General)

British Standards Institute (C T Ashton, Technical Committee Secretary)

British Veterinary Association (J H Baird, Chief Executive)

Campden Food and Drink Research Association

Centers for Disease Control, Atlanta

Clwyd Health Authority (Dr Carl Iwan Clowes, Specialist in Community Medicine)

Cold Storage and Distribution Federation (W J Bittles, Secretary General)

Commission of the European Communities (Directorates — General III and VI)

Consumers' Association

Convention of Scottish Local Authorities (Bruce Black, for Secretary General)

Co-operative Wholesale Society (Sir Dennis Landau, Mr Duncan Bowdler and Mr Gordon Amery)

Dairy Trade Federation (L J Hall, Divisional Director-Technical)

Darlington Health Authority (A Johnson, Infection Control Officer and Brian Footit, Unit General Manager, Memorial Hospital)

Dudley Road Hospital, Department of Medical Microbiology (Richard Wise, Consultant Medical Microbiologist)

East Suffolk Health Authority (Dr M F H Bush, Director of Public Health)

The Farm and Food Society (J Bower, Hon. Secretary)

Farmers Union of Wales (Mrs R Mary James, Commodities Executive Officer)

Federation of Wholesale Distributors (Alan Toft, Director General)

Food and Drink Federation (M A Hunt, Scientific & Technical Division)

Food Safety Advisory Centre (Michael Young, Executive Director)

Gateshead Health Authority (A O Sobo, Specialist in Community Medicine)

Goat Producers Association (A Mowlem, Chairman)

Institution of Environmental Health Officers (Mike Corbally, Principal Environmental Health Officer)

Institute of Food Research of the Agricultural and Food Research Council (especially Dr G Mead and Dr T Roberts)

Institute of Food Science and Technology (Richard B Ratcliffe, Chairman, Public Affairs Committee)

Institute of Meat, Educational Foundation (D W Leith, Director)

International Commission on Microbiological Specifications for Foods

Kingston and Esher Health Authority (A M Nelson, Director of Public Health/District Medical Officer)

Leeds Eastern Health Authority (Martin Schweiger, Specialist in Community Medicine, Medical Officer for Environmental Health, City of Leeds)
Leeds Western Health Authority (Professor Lacey)
Meat and Livestock Commission (G Harrington, Director of Planning & Research)
National Association of Master Bakers, Confectioners and Caterers (D W Harbourne, Director)
National Consumer Council (Maurice Healy, Director)
National Farmers' Union of Scotland (D Scott Johnson, Chief Executive)
Richard A E North (Consultant in Environmental Health and Safety)
Northumberland Health Authority (Helen Watson, District Medical Officer/Director of Public Health)
Oldham Health Authority (P M Shrigley, District General Manager)
Pontefract Health Authority (G Lumb, District Catering Manager)
The Public Health Laboratory Service
The Retail Consortium (Mrs Clare Cheney, Assistant Director-Food)
Royal College of Physicians, Faculty of Community Medicine (Miss L Frankland, Secretary)
The Royal Institute of Public Health and Hygiene (W A Wadell, Secretary)
The Royal Society of Health (R Campbell, Acting Secretary)
Sandwell Health Authority (Dr J D Middleton, Director of Public Health and Dr M R Evans, Senior Registrar in Public Health)
Society for Applied Bacteriology (Dr Dorothy Jones)
South Glamorgan Health Authority (G L Harrhy, General Manager)
Spar (UK) Ltd (John Stanton, Trading Director)
Specialist Cheesemakers Association
Thurrock Borough Council (D J Allen, Environmental Health Manager)
Transfrigoroute UK Ltd
United Kingdom Agricultural Supply Trade Association (Miss J Nelson, Manager-Feed)
United Kingdom Egg Producers Association (Keith Pulman, Secretary)
United Kingdom Dairy Association (Dr J F Gordon, Chairman — Technical Committee)
United States Food and Drugs Administration
United States Department of Agriculture
Wiltshire Food Group of Environmental Health Officers (M S Wildsmith, Convenor)
World Health Organization

We are also grateful to the various individuals in Government Departments for their contributions and to the many other individuals and companies who have willingly shown us their activities and processes, and to whom we have expressed our thanks directly.

CHAPTER 2

FOODBORNE ILLNESS: GENERAL CONCLUSIONS

THE CAUSES OF FOODBORNE ILLNESS

2.1 Throughout the work of the Committee, we have had in mind that Ministers asked us to consider why there has been a major increase in foodborne illness in the UK in recent years. Comments relevant to this appear at various places throughout both parts of our report. This section presents a synopsis.

2.2 Consideration of the matter cannot be limited to the UK alone. Foodborne illness is a common problem elsewhere, for example in other Western European countries and in the United States. Underlying causes therefore have to be considered in an international context.

2.3 We do not believe that there is any single cause of the increase. Rather there are a number of factors which have led to the present situation. We examine these in turn under the following sub-headings:—

— levels of reporting and enhanced publicity;

— terminology: sources and causes of infection;

— food sources of infection;

— causes contributing to foodborne infection, including:—

    a.   technology and its control;

    b.   changes in lifestyle and habits;

    c.   hygiene awareness;

    d.   international travel and commerce.

Levels of reporting and enhanced publicity

2.4 The United Kingdom has reporting systems which we consider to be more efficient in relation to those in other countries. We have examined them in Part I, Chapter 3, and Part II, Chapter 3. We are in no doubt that there has been a real increase in the incidence of food poisoning in recent years. The statistical series clearly show upward trends in food poisoning of different kinds (see Part I, Chapter 2 and Appendices 1, 2 and 3; and Part II, paragraph 1.18 and Chapter 3). However, the true size of these increases is difficult to assess accurately. This is because the data come from different sources which are not easily reconcilable and there is also a degree of under-reporting, the extent of which probably varies from year to year and from one type of food poisoning to another. In addition it is difficult to assess the effect that greater awareness of the upward trend in the incidence of food poisoning itself has on reporting. General practices and laboratories, realising that data on food poisoning are needed, may put more effort into making fuller returns.

2.5 In our view one of the most important tasks of the new Steering Group and Advisory Committee structure which is being set up (see Part II, paragraph 1.21 (b)) will be to undertake a thorough analysis of the extent to which the magnitude of the trends in the reported incidence of foodborne illness of various types is real or the product of more complete reporting.

2.6 Over and above the difficulty of getting an accurate and objective measure of incidence and trends in food poisoning, we believe the Steering Group and Advisory Committee structure needs to address the question of the public perception of the situation. Awareness of what is happening among the general public is much influenced by the media. In this respect food poisoning is no different from many other areas of public concern. At various points in our report we have stressed the need for understandable but authoritative official statements on the trends in various types of food poisoning. In the absence of such briefing, and to a degree because of the difficulties of analysing the reported data, misleading — and indeed alarmist — views can easily be generated. Not only is such a state of affairs undesirable from the point of view of developing a coherent policy for dealing with the situation, such perceptions may themselves have some effect on the gathering of statistics, and in particular on the level of reporting.

Terminology: sources and causes of infection

2.7 In the two parts of our report we have devoted a number of chapters to the examination of particular foods which we judged to be of most concern in relation to food poisoning. In what follows we distinguish between two concepts: the source of food poisoning; and the cause of food poisoning. The source is the place (foodstuff, environment, water, dirt, pests, etc) from which the potentially infecting microorganisms arise. Many processes used in food preparation and processing (cooking, use of preservatives, etc) block the passage of these source organisms to humans and thus prevent food poisoning. The cause is the change in circumstances or arrangements whereby the microorganisms from the source breach defences and cause illness. Among these causes are failures in equipment and in procedures, and also human error; but changes in general policy and practice (for example a general decision to market a food without customary preservatives) can also be an important cause of infection.

Food sources of infection

2.8 We see poultry and their products as the most important source of human gastrointestinal infections arising from food. Over the past forty years, the poultry industry has transformed what was a luxury meat into a cheap and plentiful source of protein, successfully bringing a wide range of new, nutritious and popular products within the price range of many households. This transformation has been achieved by greatly increasing the size of production units and the throughput of slaughterhouses and of processing plants. Infection, once introduced into a flock, can therefore now be transmitted to other birds within the flock on a far greater scale than in the past, and the nature of the slaughter process makes it inevitable that any contamination present in some birds will be further spread during processing (see Part I, paragraph 6.45). We have noted (see Part I, paragraphs 6.9 and 6.10) the high proportion of carcases contaminated with salmonella and campylobacter; and shell eggs can also be a source of salmonella.

2.9 We found red meat to be a source of microorganisms capable of causing foodborne illness, although on a much lesser scale than poultry and its products (Part II, Chapter 4). Liquid milk (Part II, Chapter 5) is a source of pathogenic microorganisms in its raw state, since it presents a very favourable medium in which they can multiply; however, it is not generally a source once it has been pasteurised or subjected to an equivalent heat treatment. There are some known problem areas where fish and shellfish can be a source of microbiological foodborne illness (see Part II, Chapter 6) — eg the propensity of some shellfish to pick up from polluted waters pathogenic viruses which are not removed by depuration.

Causes contributing to foodborne infection

a. Technology and its control

2.10 The processes involved in producing food are obviously potentially a key factor in determining whether or not pathogenic microorganisms pass from sources to people. For example, we noted in Part I, Chapter 6, that the technology and equipment currently used in poultry slaughterhouses and processing plants, coupled with the high speed of throughput, make it difficult to prevent cross-contamination of carcases: the technology and equipment may therefore be an indirect cause of food poisoning if the meat is not properly handled and cooked. This factor is far less important in relation to red meat: contact with gut contents or with the outer surface of a contaminated carcase can result in cross-contamination of animals in the abattoir, but the potential for this is far less than with poultry, since numbers are fewer, line speeds are slower, and individual carcases generally get more careful attention. In relation to liquid milk, heat treatment minimises the effect of any contamination. There is a need for care when raw untreated milk is used to prepare a product (eg soft cheese) which is not subject to processing equivalent to pasteurisation. In relation to shellfish the depuration process is effective in removing bacteria, but no process has yet been devised for reliably eliminating viruses.

2.11 Traditionally the food manufacturer has relied largely on microbiological testing of raw materials and products to ensure safety. It is now recognised that this approach is inadequate in the context of today's often highly complex food manufacturing operations. Throughout its report, the Committee has advocated the Hazard Analysis Critical Control Point approach to safety assurance, not only in manufacture, but in all sections of the food industry.

b. Changes in lifestyle and habits

2.12 The last two decades have seen some major changes in lifestyle. There has been a decline in the formal meal, and an increase in "snacking" and in eating while travelling. There is growing use of fast foods, of take-aways and of convenience foods. The food industry has responded to these changes by producing a wide range of convenience foods which call on new technologies. The currently available range of chilled foods and ready-to-cook meals was not achievable with the technological capability which existed twenty years ago. Fast food establishments, take-aways, ethnic restaurants and more traditional eating places have proliferated. All these make extensive use of frozen and chilled pre-prepared dishes. Much of this food is of excellent quality, but it needs careful storage and cooking which it does not always receive. In addition food is often made up some time before it is to be eaten; inadequate arrangements for storing the food may then cause food poisoning.

2.13 Many customers now shop at supermarkets weekly or less frequently. They rely on the home refrigerator or freezer to keep food in good condition until it is required. These practices do, however, require more care to be exercised in handling and storage, particularly in relation to foods produced by some of the newer technologies. Chilled foods, for example, may present new hazards from pathogenic bacteria capable of growing at low temperatures; hence temperature control has assumed greater importance. Greater reliance upon refrigerators also places demands both on their design and capabilities and on the way that people use them.

2.14 Another aspect of changing lifestyles is the growing public concern with what are seen as artificial or 'unhealthy' components of manufactured foods. This concern has led to the reduction or removal of ingredients, such as preservatives, which have in the past played an important role in preventing the growth of pathogenic bacteria in food.

2.15 As noted in paragraph 2.8 above, a particular change in eating habits in recent years has been the rise of poultry meat as a regular item in the family diet. In view of the importance of poultry as a source of infection (see paragraph 2.8 above and Part I, Chapter 6), we consider it incontrovertible that the increase in poultry meat consumption over recent years is one contributory factor underlying the rise in salmonella and campylobactor infections. UK production of poultry meat rose from an average of 744,000 tonnes deadweight in 1978-80 to 1,048,000 tonnes in 1988 — an increase of 41%. Given that handling and preparation will not always be perfect, the popularity of poultry meat must in our view be associated with the increased incidence of food poisoning.

c. Hygiene awareness

2.16 We have found that a lack of understanding of the basic principles of microbiology and of food hygiene has been a contributory factor where problems have arisen over the microbiological safety of food. This is the case throughout the food chain: we have seen examples of such lack of understanding on the part of farmers, manufacturers, wholesalers, retailers, caterers and consumers. Training and education are of the highest importance. We have seen shortcomings amongst managers, who are directly responsible for an effective training programme which will ensure the safety of their product; amongst those responsible for the enforcement of the legislation, notably EHOs; and at home and at school, where the understanding of food hygiene starts. We therefore believe that the lack of effective training and education is an important factor underlying the current levels of foodborne illness. We expand on this in Part II, Chapter 11.

d. International travel and commerce

2.17 International travel and trade are already important routes by which infection is spread. Travel and trade have increased steadily over recent years and this is likely to continue.

GENERAL CONCLUSIONS 2.18 In summary, therefore, we see the present level of foodborne illness in the UK as reflecting many different causes and as part of an international problem. Factors relevant in increasing the risk of foodborne illness range from changes in agricultural practice, changes in the pattern of food consumption, changes in the way food is processed and handled and changes in the lifestyle of consumers. No one of these areas is predominent: no one category of participants in the food chain has sole blame or sole responsibility. All those involved in the food chain have their part to play in minimising the risks.

2.19 The opportunities available have stimulated the food industry to produce new products and to develop new technologies, always under competition. The industry has responded vigorously to this challenge with the result that in this country we now have a wide selection of foods at competitive prices. However, any development in the technology of food supply brings with it the need to assess rigorously the implications for food safety. We intend that our report should contribute to this process, and thus ensure the establishment of a proper balance between the requirements of convenience and of food safety.

CHAPTER 3

SCOTLAND AND NORTHERN IRELAND

3.1 Many of the matters dealt with in Chapters 6, 7 and 8 of Part I, and those relating to the rest of the food chain in Chapters 4 to 10 of this part of the report, apply equally to Scotland and Northern Ireland as to England and Wales.

3.2 This chapter discusses the particular organisation in Scotland and Northern Ireland for collecting data on foodborne illness and discusses the trends in foodborne illness compared with those for England and Wales. It deals with the arrangements for the surveillance of food and of food animals which are specific to Scotland and Northern Ireland and compares them with those in England and Wales. It also considers the liaison arrangements between health, animal health and food interests.

3.3 The populations of Scotland and Northern Ireland are much smaller than that of England, even Scotland being no greater in size than a single English health region. For this reason the statistics, particularly those for Northern Ireland, are more likely to be subject to variation because of relatively infrequent events such as outbreaks.

SCOTLAND

ORGANISATION OF HEALTH SERVICES AND LOCAL AUTHORITY ENVIRONMENTAL HEALTH SERVICES IN SCOTLAND

3.4 The population of Scotland is about 5.1 million, which is around one-tenth of the population of England and Wales. Just under one-third live in the three cities of Glasgow, Edinburgh and Aberdeen. The area of Scotland is slightly over half that of England and Wales and consequently population density outside the main cities is low compared with England and Wales, particularly in the Highlands and Islands.

3.5 The Secretary of State for Scotland, acting through the Scottish Home and Health Department (SHHD), is ultimately responsible for the National Health Service in Scotland which is administered by 15 Health Boards. This differs from the systems operating in England and Wales. In England the functions of the Secretary of State for Health are carried out by 14 Regional and 190 District Health Authorities whilst in Wales the Secretary of State for Wales is responsible for the nine District Health Authorities. In Scotland, as in Wales, there is no administrative tier equivalent to the Regional Health Authority. In functional terms a Health Board in Scotland may be considered as generally equivalent to Regional and District Health Authorities and Family Health Services Authorities in England.

3.6 Mainland Scotland is divided into nine local government regions which in turn are further divided into a total of 53 local government districts. There are also three all-purpose Islands Councils. With the exception of the Strathclyde Region, which includes four Health Boards, each Regional and Islands Council is coterminous with a Health Board, which is helpful in allowing effective joint management by Local Authorities and Health Boards of problems of food safety. These arrangements are more satisfactory than in parts of England where there are boundary problems to which we have previously referred (Part I, paragraphs 4.11-4.12). Each of the Islands and Districts has a Director of Environmental Health (or equivalent) with responsibility for enforcement in respect of food safety.

3.7 The Common Services Agency (CSA) for the National Health Service in Scotland provides several important centrally administered services. These services include the Information and Statistics Division (ISD), which collates and analyses health service related information for Scotland, and publishes an annual summary of returns of notifiable diseases including food poisoning. The Information and Statistics Division therefore, in this context, performs a function equivalent to that of the Office of Population Censuses and Surveys (OPCS) in England and Wales.

3.8 The Communicable Diseases (Scotland) Unit (CD(S)U), located at Ruchill Hospital, Glasgow, is another Division of the Common Services Agency. It is broadly analogous to the Communicable Disease Surveillance Centre (CDSC) in England and Wales. The CD(S)U is a multi-disciplinary unit of 28 staff drawn from the disciplines of epidemiology, clinical medicine, microbiology, nursing, environmental health and veterinary medicine. Its functions include surveillance of infection in Scotland, co-ordination of relevant organisations in the investigation and control of infection, dissemination of information on infection, advising SHHD on infection problems, and teaching and training. CD(S)U also carries out the epidemiological analysis of communicable disease statistics including food poisoning.

3.9 The CD(S)U has close links with, but is not directly related to, any laboratories. This differs from the situation in England and Wales where CDSC is an integral part of the PHLS and therefore has right of access to and support from all the laboratories of the PHLS. There is no analogue of the PHLS in Scotland.

3.10 A microbiological laboratory service for public health is provided in Scotland by health board and university laboratories as and when needed. However, SHHD funds centrally some health board laboratories and one university laboratory to act as reference laboratories including the Scottish Salmonella Reference Laboratory at Stobhill General Hospital, Glasgow. Health board and university laboratories in Scotland also use the services of the Central Public Health Laboratory (CPHL), Colindale, in some circumstances (see paragraph 3.16).

SOURCES OF INFORMATION ON HUMAN ILLNESS

3.11 In Scotland, routine information on sporadic cases of human foodborne illness comes mainly from statutory notifications and from laboratory reports including those from reference laboratories in Scotland, and occasionally from the CPHL of the PHLS in England, to which samples may be referred. Additional information may also be obtained from environmental health officers, consultants in public health medicine and, occasionally, nurses and clinicians.

3.12 Information on outbreaks is reported to CD(S)U by consultants in public health medicine, by microbiologists, by consultant physicians in infectious diseases and by environmental health officers of local authorities. This is similar to England and Wales (see Part I, Chapter 3).

Statutory Notifications

3.13 In Scotland the statutory notification of some diseases has been required since 1889. Present notifiable diseases are listed in Annex 3.1. The current legislation, the Food and Drugs (Scotland) Act 1956 and the Public Health (Notification of Infectious Diseases) (Scotland) Regulations 1988, is comparable to that prevailing in England and Wales. Medical practitioners attending patients whom they consider may be suffering from food poisoning have a statutory duty to notify the Director of Public Health/Chief Administrative Medical Officer of the Health Board for the area or his representative. Laboratory confirmation is not required but may be available in some cases. Each week the Health Boards report to the ISD of the CSA (see paragraph 3.7) the number of cases of food poisoning of which they are aware. Unlike in England and Wales, these reports do not distinguish between statutorily notified cases and additional cases which become known by means other than formal notification. The Scottish reports, therefore, appear to be equivalent in England and Wales to formal notifications plus those "ascertained by other means". They do not provide information on whether the food poisoning was thought to be contracted at home or abroad. The Information and Statistics Division (ISD) routinely passes this information on to SHHD and to CD(S)U. CD(S)U publishes data on notifiable diseases in the Communicable Diseases (Scotland) Weekly Report together with information on reportable infections (see paragraph 3.17) and other laboratory reports (see paragraph 3.15). The ISD of the CSA also publishes an annual summary in a report entitled "Scottish Health Statistics". Further details on publications may be found in paragraphs 3.25 to 3.27. The above differences between Scotland, and England and Wales, in the information collected and in its collation and reporting, make direct comparison of data between the countries difficult. We comment on the need for compatibility of data throughout the UK in paragraph 3.38.

3.14 In the absence of a statutory definition of food poisoning anywhere in the United Kingdom, as noted in Part I, Scotland has used since 1980 the World Health Organization (WHO) definition: "any disease of an infectious or toxic nature caused by or thought to be caused by the consumption of food or water." We recommend in Part I, paragraph 3.49, that guidelines on the case definition of food poisoning should be developed so as to assist uniformity of notifying practices. **We further recommend that Government should work towards a common definition of food poisoning for all countries of the United Kingdom, and ideally for the whole of the European Community** (R(II)3.1).

Laboratory reports

3.15 Since 1967 all National Health Service (NHS) and university microbiology laboratories in Scotland have voluntarily reported laboratory diagnosed infections to CD(S)U. This is similar to the position in England and Wales but from evidence received we gathered that reporting may be more complete than in NHS laboratories south of the border.

3.16 Further detailed information on microorganisms is obtained from reference laboratories in Scotland, in particular the Scottish Salmonella Reference Laboratory in Glasgow which reports its results directly to CD(S)U. Samples are sent to CPHL in suspected cases of botulism, and for phage typing and/or toxin testing of *S. typhi*, *S. paratyphi* and other enterobacteria such as Yersinia, Aeromonas and Verocytotoxin producing *E. coli*, listeria, *Staphylococcus aureus* and *Bacillus* species. The results of these investigations are reported to the originating laboratory.

Reportable Infections

3.17 Since 1989 the laboratory reporting system has been strengthened by the identification of 30 formally designated "reportable infections" on which information is specifically sought. This is a non-statutory administrative arrangement to encourage the collection of as much information as possible on these infections which are quite distinct from the "notifiable diseases" referred to in paragraph 3.13 above. Although, in practice, laboratories provide the bulk of the information, EHOs, consultants in public health medicine, nurses and clincians are encouraged to provide information on the reportable infections to CD(S)U. The list of reportable infections (Annex 3.2) includes infections which are transmissible by food such as salmonellosis, campylobacter infection, listeriosis and *E. coli* 0157 infection. This arrangement provides flexibility and readily permits diseases to be added or removed from the list as circumstances change. We welcome this.

National Surveillance Co-ordinators

3.18 There is a group of "national surveillance coordinators" (NSCs) each of whom has interest and expertise in a particular "reportable infection". The NSC may be a doctor, environmental health officer or veterinarian acting on a voluntary part-time basis in addition to their other duties and reporting informally to the Director of CD(S)U. They take responsiblity for investigating the epidemiology of a particular reportable infection, not only in the area in which they work, but throughout Scotland. They are expected to produce an annual report. Since the system is voluntary the NSCs have no contractual obligation to report to any particular authority, but have frequent contacts with CD(S)U staff. When it is considered advisable to follow up cases, or to obtain further information, the NSCs will contact the reporting laboratory and, if necessary, visit and discuss relevant cases with the microbiologist and clinician. They can also assist the local consultant in public health medicine to carry out further studies when indicated.

3.19 The Committee noted that no extra resources had generally been provided for the NSCs who were expected to carry out this role in addition to their main full-time appointments. We believe that the NSCs are carrying out important functions. **We therefore recommend to the Scottish Office that the current arrangements for national surveillance coordinators should be placed on a more formal basis with any necessary expenses being met and an obligation to report to the Director of CD(S)U at least annually** (R(II)3.2).

General Practice spotter schemes

3.20 We have described in Part I, paragraph 3.18, the Royal College of General Practitioners (RCGP) sentinel practice scheme which covers a wide range of diagnoses including infectious intestinal disease. Unfortunately there are no longer any Scottish practices taking part in this scheme. There is, however, a group of 124 "spotter" practices, covering 657,000 people in 11 out of 15 Health Boards, which has developed since 1971 specifically for the surveillance of influenza. We understand that consideration is being given to linking the 124 practices together in the development of an existing electronic network and to extending the range of diseases reported. **We recommend to the Scottish Home and Health Department that the proposed linking together of general practices through the development of an existing electronic network should proceed and that infectious gastrointestinal disease be included in the diseases reported** (R(II)3.3).

3.21 We have noted in Part II, paragraph 1.21(a), that a pilot scheme for a national survey of infectious gastrointestinal diseases based on general practices is being planned in England and Wales. **We recommend that the Steering Group on the Microbiological Safety of Food should consider including general practices from other countries of the United Kingdom in any subsequent plans for a nationwide survey of infectious gastrointestinal disease** (R(II)3.4).

Sources of information on outbreaks

3.22 The Chief Medical Officer is required to be informed immediately of any serious outbreak of foodborne disease, as is the case in England and in Wales. Outbreaks of foodborne disease are investigated and reported to CD(S)U on standard outbreak summary forms by consultants in public health medicine and environmental health officers and earlier details are frequently relayed by telephone or as preliminary reports. Additionally, a parallel laboratory system reports outbreaks or sporadic cases of foodborne disease where a microorganism or toxin has been identified. These arrangements seem to work satisfactorily and, although some household outbreaks may escape the reporting mechanism, it is unlikely that general community or institutional outbreaks are unreported. Thus, reporting of outbreaks seems to be broadly similar to that in England and Wales. Scotland uses the same definition of an outbreak as that used in England and Wales (see Part I, paragraph 3.20).

Food Hazard Warnings

The SHHD issues "hazard warnings" to EHOs and to consultants in public health medicine drawing attention to foodborne hazards. These are usually distributed to environmental health departments, directors of public health and food and dairy officers. These "hazard warnings" may be issued jointly with other Health Departments of the United Kingdom depending on how the hazard is distributed.

Guidance on the management of outbreaks

3.24 The Committee has seen the draft of a handbook, entitled "The investigation and control of foodborne and waterborne disease in Scotland", giving guidance to the Scottish Health Service on the handling of outbreaks. We understand it will be issued shortly. In Part I we pointed out the need for a code of practice giving guidance on the management of outbreaks, and recommended that the Steering Group on the Microbiological Safety of Food should give early attention to the need to produce such a code. If the constituent countries of the UK produce their own guidance we believe that it is of the greatest importance that the Steering Group ensures that there is a consistency of approach among countries.

Publication of information

3.25 The "Weekly Report" published by CD(S)U contains details of notifiable diseases, of reportable infections and of isolations of zoonotic organisms from animals (see paragraph 3.46). It is available to those involved in the control of infections eg NHS, veterinary and local authority environmental health staff. In Part I, paragraphs 3.44-3.45, we stated that wide dissemination of information on the microbiological contamination of food was important. We consider therefore that the "Weekly Report" should be publicly available.

3.26 The Registrar General for Scotland publishes a four-weekly digest of statistics on infectious diseases, including food poisoning, based on information supplied from ISD, entitled "Vital Statistics Returns of the Registrar General for Scotland".

3.27 CD(S)U and the Scottish Salmonella Reference Laboratory have published since 1970 an annual report entitled "Salmonellosis in Scotland". This report contains relevant information from the Weekly Reports and elsewhere about salmonella isolates from human, veterinary and other sources. Since 1980 CD(S)U and ISD have also published annually a wider ranging report, called "Surveillance programme for foodborne infections and intoxications — Scotland", as part of the WHO Surveillance Programme for the Control of Foodborne Infections and Intoxications in Europe.

TRENDS IN FOODBORNE ILLNESS IN SCOTLAND

3.28 The reporting of most gastrointestinal pathogens by laboratories in Scotland to CD(S)U (Figure 3.1A) showed trends in the 1980s essentially similar to those observed in England and Wales (see Part I, Figure 2.2), but there were notable differences in trends in salmonellas, particularly when these were expressed as rates per 100,000 population.

3.29 There were also marked differences between the notification rates for food poisoning in Scotland and the formal notification rates in England and Wales especially up until the late 1980's; those for the years 1975 to 1989 for both Scotland and England and Wales are shown with numbers and mid-year populations in Table 3.1, and in Figure 3.2. In England and Wales formal notification rates increased steadily from 18.0 per 100,000 in 1975 to 26.6 per 100,000 in 1984, followed by a nearly three-fold increase to over 75 per 100,000 population in 1989. The Scottish data showed a different pattern; notification rates were around twice those of England and Wales in the late 1970's, increased to a peak of over 56 per 100,000 in 1981, declined in the mid 1980's, and rose again almost in parallel with the rates in England and Wales but reaching a lower level of nearly 63 per 100,000 in 1989. The rate in Scotland in 1989 was only a little above that observed in the previous peak in 1981, whereas the rate for England and Wales in 1989 was more than three times that of 1981.

3.30 Laboratory reports to CD(S)U of salmonella isolates in Scotland for the years 1975-1989 are shown in Table 3.2A. Reports to CDSC are shown in Table 3.2C. The rates per 100,000 population are compared with those for England and Wales in Figures 3.3, 3.4 and 3.5. The rates for all salmonellas follow the general pattern of statutory notifications, but the large difference observed between statutory notification rates for food poisoning in Scotland and those in England and Wales in the late 1970's was not present (Figure 3.3). The peak of notifications and laboratory reports observed in Scotland in the early 1980's was due to a rise in reports of *S. typhimurium* and was seen in England and Wales at a proportionately lower level and a year later (Figure 3.4). This was attributed mainly to bovine infection (see Part I, Appendix 1, paragraph A1.13). The rise in the late 1980's in both Scotland and England and Wales was due to *S. enteritidis* (Figure 3.5), although this rise began slightly earlier in Scotland (1981) than in England and Wales (1983). In Scotland, as in England and Wales, the rise was mainly in *S. enteritidis* phage type 4 and was largely associated with infection in poultry.

3.31 The differences in notification rates between Scotland and England and Wales have not been satisfactorily explained. More complete notification could partly account for the higher rates in Scotland in the 1970's, although no information is available on the completeness of notification by medical practitioners in Scotland compared with England and Wales. The fact that the notification data for Scotland include other cases of food poisoning of which Health Boards are aware, in addition to formally notified cases, may explain some of the difference and this is supported by the data collected in England and Wales since 1982 of formal notifications plus cases ascertained by other means (Figure 3.2). However, since 1986 the annual rates of total food poisoning in England and Wales have exceeded the notification rates in Scotland at the time of the *S. enteritidis* epidemic, although this difference was not reflected in laboratory reports of *S. enteritidis* (Figure 3.5). Other factors that may be relevant in explaining apparent differences in reported rates of food poisoning include the relative absence of *S. hadar* from turkey meat in Scotland compared with England and Wales, the ban on the sale of raw cows milk introduced in Scotland in 1983 and the proportionately greater epidemic of *S. typhimurium* in the early 1980's referred to in paragraph 3.30 above.

3.32 Campylobacter infections rose considerably in Scotland in the 1980's (Table 3.3); in 1988 the number of laboratory reports (2,906) exceeded those of salmonellas (2,580). However, unlike the data on statutory notifications of food poisoning and on laboratory reports of salmonellas, the pattern of campylobacter infections was similar in Scotland and in England and Wales; the rise during the 1980's, expressed as rates per 100,000 population, was almost identical (Figure 3.6).

3.33 Reported cases of listeriosis increased in Scotland between 1980 and 1988 as they did in England and Wales (Table 3.4) and then declined in 1989.

Information on Outbreaks 3.34 Table 3.5 sets out the overall number of outbreaks and number of people involved for 1980-1988 (unclassified by aetiological agent). These relate to household and general community/institutional outbreaks. Table 3.6 gives details by type of outbreak and aetiological agent for 1988. Full details are published in the annual report "Surveillance programme for foodborne infections and intoxications in Scotland".

3.35 In 1988 there were 155 outbreaks in Scotland due to salmonellas of which 41 were general outbreaks and 114 household outbreaks. In England and Wales 455 outbreaks were recorded in the same year, a proportionally lower figure when allowance is made for the difference in population size. In 1989 computerisation of laboratory reported data in England and Wales at CDSC permitted more readily the linkage of cases in patients with the same surname; as a result the number of recorded family outbreaks rose and the total outbreaks reported nearly doubled from 455 in 1988 to 955 in 1989. This suggests that some of the difference in recorded outbreaks between Scotland and England and Wales in earlier years may have been due to difficulties in England and Wales of linking sporadic cases manually when dealing with much larger numbers than in Scotland.

3.36 Table 3.7 shows all the general community and institutional outbreaks due to salmonellas between 1986 and 1989 which originated in Scotland and the suspected food vehicles. In over 70% of general outbreaks the food vehicle was identified. Similar information on food vehicles in household outbreaks was not available.

3.37 In outbreaks due to *Bacillus cereus, Clostridium perfringens* and *Staphylococcus aureus* the food vehicle is identified more frequently than in outbreaks due to salmonellas (Appendix 4, Table A4.1). Residual food is more likely to be available for examination in outbreaks where the illness has a short incubation period.

Compatibility of data

3.38 In Part I, paragraph 3.51, we recommend that Government encourage the standardisation of data collection and reporting of food poisoning microorganisms internationally and in particular throughout the European Community as soon as possible. It is important, therefore, that the constituent countries of the UK also ensure, as far as possible, compatibility of their data. We believe there needs to be agreement on the case-definition of food poisoning, on methods of collating and reporting data and on the precise choice of denominators when calculating rates. A recommendation to this effect is contained in paragraph 1.19 above.

LABORATORY FUNDING/ORGANISATION

3.39 Since an organisation equivalent to the PHLS does not exist in Scotland, public health work that is normally done in PHLS laboratories in England and Wales is carried out by NHS hospital laboratories in Scotland. Under current arrangements, apart from central funding for reference laboratories (see paragraph 3.10), we understand that no budget is provided specifically to cover public health work in Scottish NHS laboratories. A single budget for all purposes is assigned to each laboratory by the relevant Health Board and the costs of public health work are met from this general budget as and when the need arises. The Committee is concerned that in any laboratory, whose main purpose is the care of individual patients, public health work is liable to take second place whenever the clinical workload mounts. We are also concerned that public health work might take second place when funding is limited. Nor do we believe that the informal method of working, which has operated in the past, is compatible with the provisions of the NHS and Community Care Act 1990 under which work undertaken could be the subject of contractual arrangements. **The Committee therefore recommends that the Scottish Home and Health Department should identify and fund a core group of laboratories explicitly to undertake public health microbiological work** (R(II)3.5).

FOOD SURVEILLANCE

3.40 A Scottish Food Coordinating Committee (SFCC) was set up in 1983 for two purposes; first, to coordinate enforcement effort through discussions of difficult points of legal interpretation and second, to act as a focus for the local liaison groups described in paragraph 3.48 below. Membership of the SFCC consists of public analysts, directors of environmental health, representatives of SHHD, DAFS and Local Authority Coordinating Body on Trading Standards (LACOTS), a bacteriologist and other specialists as necessary. It covers both chemical and microbiological hazards in food.

3.41 The SFCC may initiate special surveys or projects through its Working Party on Food Surveillance. Some 31 projects have been initiated to date of which only four were specifically concerned with the microbiological safety of food. This committee can play a useful role in coordinating or undertaking microbiological surveillance in Scotland. **We recommend that the Steering Group on the Microbiological Safety of Food should liaise with the Scottish Food Coordinating Committee on the surveillance of the microbiological safety of food in Scotland** (R(II)3.6).

ORGANISATION OF VETERINARY SERVICES IN SCOTLAND

3.42 In Scotland, responsibilities for veterinary matters having a bearing on the protection of public health are not organised in the same way as in England and Wales:—

— In England and Wales, a veterinary diagnostic service is provided by the nineteen Veterinary Investigation Centres (VICs) which comprise the Veterinary Investigation Service (VIS) (an arm of the SVS). A similar function is performed by the eight Scottish VICs: however, these form one of the Divisions of the Scottish Agriculture College system (SAC). The SAC is a body which is funded by the DAFS in respect of educational, research and development and certain advisory services, and which is also required to generate income from commercial sources;

— In England and Wales the local Senior Veterinary Investigation Officers (who work within the VIS) are nominated to receive the notifications of isolations of salmonella that must be made under the Zoonoses Order 1989. In Scotland the nominated officers are the Divisional Veterinary Officers (DVOs) (who work in the Veterinary Field Service of the SVS), reflecting the fact that the Veterinary Investigation Service of the SVS does not operate in Scotland;

— On both sides of the border, the nominated officer is responsible for arranging follow-up action when notifications are received. In Scotland, this includes the prompt notification of the relevant Consultant in Public Health Medicine by the DVO. In the case of invasive salmonellae, new serotypes, or where there is a likelihood of humans being affected, the DVO will organise an investigation on the farm. Serotyping will already have taken place at the SVS's Lasswade laboratory (which in this respect fulfils the role played by the Central Veterinary Laboratory (CVL) in England and Wales). If it is considered that further samples must be tested they will be sent to the appropriate SAC VIC. In the case of other salmonellas, the DVO may initiate an investigation on the farm and any samples collected on that visit will also be sent to the appropriate VIC. This again parallels the arrangements in England and Wales, though the fact that the Scottish VICs are within the SAC system means that the funding arrangements are different; the SAC receives a block grant from DAFS to enable it to do this work.

3.43 The Scottish arrangements are therefore complex by comparison with those which apply in England and Wales. The State Veterinary Service is involved in both cases, but in Scotland there is additional involvement on the part of the SAC — an independent agency — and the Scottish Office, which funds the relevant SAC activities and is answerable to the Secretary of State in respect of his responsibility for providing in Scotland the veterinary services which the law requires to be provided. In this context we were informed in particular that the Assistant Chief Veterinary Officer who heads the SVS in Scotland, as well as reporting to the Chief Veterinary Officer (CVO) in London, is responsible for advising the Secretary of State for Scotland.

3.44 We considered whether arrangements of such complexity actually worked effectively. All the evidence we received suggests that this is the case. However, we wonder whether coordination would remain effective under the pressure of a large outbreak involving animals and the human population. **We recommend that the**

Government keep the arrangements for veterinary microbiology related to food safety in Scotland under review (R(II)3.7).

Surveillance of food animals and publication of results

3.45 One series of data on the incidence of salmonella and brucella organisms in farm animals is provided — in Scotland as in England and Wales — by the statutory notifications received by the SVS under the Zoonoses Order 1989. These data are published annually in the report entitled "Salmonellosis in Scotland" which, as described in paragraph 3.27, reviews all isolations of salmonellas in Scotland reported to CD(S)U by both medical and veterinary laboratories including additional information from the Scottish Salmonella Reference Laboratory and the Division of Enteric Pathogens, PHLS, Colindale.

3.46 In addition, reports of isolations of zoonotic organisms (see Annex 3.3) by the VIC's of the SAC are sent every week directly to CD(S)U for inclusion in the Weekly Reports, and to the CVL at Weybridge for inclusion in the VIDA system (see Part I, paragraph 3.29). The data gathered in this way cover only those cases where private veterinary surgeons have felt it necessary to call for laboratory analyses as a diagnostic aid. Even though by its nature incomplete, the central collection of such data is useful in identifying trends in the incidence of pathogens in animals. As mentioned in paragraph 3.25, the isolations from animals are also published in CD(S)U's Weekly Report. Thus the system in Scotland works more promptly than the system in England and Wales in collating health information from human and veterinary sources and provides a picture of the current state of the microbiological contamination of humans and food animals and of any developing trends. We welcome these arrangements and we feel that similar arrangements should be considered in England and Wales in relation to our recommendations in Part I, paragraph 3.41, on the collation of information from human and veterinary sources.

RELATIONSHIPS BETWEEN VETERINARY AND MEDICAL STAFF

3.47 All information about isolates of zoonotic organisms in animals which comes to the DVO is promptly passed to the relevant Consultant in Public Health Medicine and to the Director of Environmental Health in the relevant local authority district as noted in paragraph 3.42 above. Good central liaison between the veterinary staff involved and the CD(S)U is also vital if the public health implications of zoonoses are to be properly assessed and dealt with, especially in acute situations. Liaison with the CD(S)U is specified as a responsibility of one of the Senior Veterinary Officer posts in the SVS's headquarters office in Edinburgh. Until recently, day to day liaison work was carried out by a Veterinary Officer of the SVS, who in discharge of this function spent 40% of his time at the CD(S)U at Ruchill Hospital. The CD(S)U itself has recently placed greater emphasis on the veterinary aspects of public health within its own organisation and the Common Services Agency has created a new post of Consultant in Veterinary Public Health, part of whose functions is to work for CD(S)U. We welcome this initiative to build veterinary knowledge and expertise into the structure of the CD(S)U. However, we would stress that this appointment does not lessen the importance of the liaison maintained with CD(S)U by the SVS. **We recommend that the State Veterinary Service maintains arrangements which properly recognise the importance of continuing liaison with the Communicable Diseases (Scotland) Unit** (R(II)3.8).

Coordination between the disciplines involved at the local level.

3.48 Local liaison groups link the medical, veterinary and environmental health disciplines within each Health Board area. They meet at least twice yearly. The local SVS, VIC, public health physicians and environmental health officers are represented at a senior level. There are also representatives of local medical and veterinary practices and a hospital microbiologist. These groups allow a regular exchange of information among the disciplines concerned and help to ensure that appropriate action is taken when necessary concerning any point in the food chain from animal to ultimate consumer. The Committee considers that such liaison groups can help establish good communication at this important interface between human and animal health.

3.49 In relation to outbreaks, we take the view that the Consultant in Public Health Medicine should be the person explicitly charged with leading and co-ordinating the response to food poisoning outbreaks at local level. The occupant of this post is equivalent to the Consultant in Communicable Disease Control whom we recommend should play this role in England and Wales (Part I, paragraph 4.44).

Coordination between disciplines involved centrally

3.50 The Committee sees a need for central coordination of the various interests concerned in the public health aspects of zoonoses and of the microbiological safety of food in Scotland. **The Committee recommends that the Scottish Office should set up a formal central group to ensure close liaison between health, animal health and food interests and to coordinate arrangements for the oversight and management of microbiological food safety matters** (R(II)3.9).

3.51 **The Committee also recommends that the central group proposed in R(II)3.9 should be closely linked with the newly established UK Steering Group on the Microbiological Safety of Food (see Part II paragraph 1.13) which has representation from Scotland** (R(II)3.10).

INFORMATION

3.52 We have already commented on the Weekly and Annual Reports published by CD(S)U. We emphasised in Part I, paragraph 3.45, the need for simple and informative briefings to the public and media at appropriate intervals. We note that more information of this sort is now being produced especially in the Food Safety Bulletin (MAFF) and Health Trends (DH). **We recommend that the relevant UK Departments consider the need for simple and informative briefings to the public and media at appropriate intervals and should ensure that the information issued to the public and the media is consistent** (R(II)3.11).

NORTHERN IRELAND

ORGANISATION OF HEALTH AND PERSONAL SOCIAL SERVICES IN NORTHERN IRELAND

3.54 Northern Ireland has a population of 1.58 million, about half of which lives in or near greater Belfast, and an area of 5,460 square miles. In terms of population the province is therefore about 3% the size of England and Wales and about 30% the size of Scotland. Its largest industry is agriculture which is a major source of trade with Great Britain and the remainder of the EC.

3.55 The Health and Personal Social Services (NI) Order 1972 places a duty on the Department of Health and Social Services Northern Ireland (DHSS(NI)) to provide, or secure the provision of, integrated health services and personal social services in Northern Ireland. The Order required the setting up of Health and Social Services Area Boards which, at the direction of DHSS(NI), are responsible as its agents for the planning, management and delivery of services in defined geographical areas.

3.56 There are four Area Boards, Eastern (645,000 population), Southern (291,000), Northern (385,000) and Western (260,000), which are broadly comparable to District Health Authorities in England, although generally larger in terms of budgets and staff. As in Scotland and Wales there is no organisational tier equivalent to the regional tier in England.

3.57 Northern Ireland is divided into 26 local government districts. The 25 District Councils outside Belfast have formed four "group" Public Health Committees, each "group" corresponding to a Health Board area, to employ EHOs. This arrangement allows the employment of specialist EHOs, including those with particular knowledge in food matters, whose expertise is available to all districts. However, because of its size, Belfast City Council, in the Eastern Health Board area, employs its own specialist EHOs. The local authority "groups" are coterminous in area with Health Board Areas except in the Eastern Health Board Area where Belfast City Council is separate from the Eastern "group". Enforcement of food legislation (currently the Food (NI) Order 1989, but to be succeeded next year by a proposed Food Safety (NI) Order 1991) is the responsibility of District Councils through their EHOs. They liaise closely with the Director of Public Health and Consultants in Public Health Medicine of the Health Boards on whom they rely for medical advice.

3.58 The Registrar General's Office for Northern Ireland has the function of collecting, collating and publishing population and vital statistics for the province, and of publishing quarterly returns of notifiable diseases including food poisoning. In these respects it is equivalent to the OPCS in England and Wales.

3.59 There is no organisation equivalent to CDSC or to CD(S)U in Northern Ireland. The analogous function is carried out by a medical division in DHSS(NI) supported by the Regional Communicable Disease Liaison Group (RCDLG) which is chaired by a senior medical officer from DHSS(NI). The RCDLG has the following functions within the province:—

i. epidemiological surveillance of communicable disease and food poisoning;

ii. collection and collation of relevant information;

iii. advice to DHSS(NI) and other Departments on policy matters relating to communicable disease control;

iv. coordination of services involved in the control of communicable disease. (Initial action in the event of an outbreak falls to the staff of the Area Health Boards. The regional coordination function comes into play in case of a serious outbreak affecting more than one Board or having possible consequences outside Northern Ireland.)

3.60 The RCDLG includes microbiologists, consultants in infectious disease, the Chief Environmental Health Officer of Department of the Environment (NI) (DOE (NI)), a Deputy Chief Veterinary Officer of the Department of Agriculture for Northern Ireland (DANI), a Nursing Officer of DHSS(NI) and the Consultant in Communicable Disease Control from each Area Health Board.

3.61 There is no Public Health Laboratory Service in Northern Ireland. No laboratory is funded specifically for public health work and there is no designated and centrally funded microbiology reference laboratory. Samples from humans are investigated at the hospital nearest to where they arise and are referred, if necssary either to the Belfast City Hospital or to the Central Public Health Laboratory Colindale, for further study.

3.62 All samples of food taken for examination by EHOs anywhere in the province are sent for examination to the Belfast City Hospital which, in this respect, has a function similar to that of the Public Health Laboratory Service in England and Wales. There is no specific funding identified for this purpose but the overall budget provided to the Eastern Health Board by DHSS(NI) is adjusted to reflec this activity. **We recommend to DHSS(NI) that the relevant allocation for the microbiological examination of foods by the Belfast City Hospital is clearly identified in the overall budget provided to the Eastern Health Board** (R(II)3.12).

**SOURCES OF
INFORMATION ON
HUMAN ILLNESS**

3.63 In Northern Ireland routine information on sporadic cases of human foodborne illness comes from statutory notifications and from voluntary reporting by laboratories to DHSS(NI).

3.64 Information on outbreaks may be reported to DHSS(NI) by consultants in public health medicine, by consultants in infectious disease and by EHOs, but there is no systematic recording of such outbreaks (see paragraph 3.70 below).

Statutory Notifications

3.65 Although food poisoning is a notifiable disease under the Public Health Act (Northern Ireland) 1967, the term has not been defined in legislation. However, a definition is given in the booklet published by DHSS(NI) in 1988 entitled "Memorandum on the Investigation and Control of Food Poisoning and Gastroenteritis in the Community". This booklet has been widely distributed to Health Boards and to EHOs in Northern Ireland. We note that Northern Ireland uses a different definition of food poisoning from that used in Scotland. England and Wales has no definition. As recorded elsewhere in our Report (paragraphs 3.14, 3.38 and 3.81) **we recommend that the Government should work towards a common definition of food poisoning for the whole of the UK** (R(II)3.13).

3.66 Doctors attending patients suffering from food poisoning in Northern Ireland are required to inform the Director of Public Health (DPH) of their local Area Health Board. The numbers of cases thus notified in each Area Board are forwarded weekly to the Regional Information Branch (RIB) of DHSS(NI). These are reported in turn to the Registrar General of Northern Ireland who publishes quarterly and yearly figures for the province. The notifications provide information on the number of cases, but not on the organisms causing illness nor on the food vehicle. As in England and Wales and Scotland they are based on clinical diagnosis.

3.67 During the investigation of outbreaks public health doctors or EHOs may detect cases of food poisoning which have not already been statutorily notified. Information on these further cases is also sent to the RIB and these data are then added to the number of statutorily notified cases without any distinction being made. So, although there is no category in the returns of "ascertained by other means" (which there is in England and Wales but not in Scotland — see paragraph 3.13) the Northern Ireland data appear to be equivalent to the England and Wales data for cases formally notified plus those "ascertained by other means". This is similar to the situation in Scotland. No information is formally collected in Northern Ireland as to whether food poisoning was contracted abroad. This is another example of differences that currently exist between the countries in the UK on the collection, collation and reporting of information. We have already commented in paragraph 3.38 above on the need for compatibility of data throughout the UK.

Laboratory reports

3.68 Reports of laboratory-confirmed human infections which may be of food origin are reported voluntarily by the province's 18 hospital laboratories to DHSS(NI). These data are equivalent to the laboratory reports to CDSC in England and Wales and to CD(S)U in Scotland. The Northern Ireland hospital laboratories also send copies of their reports to the CDSC, Colindale. There is no formal list of "reportable" human infections as there is in Scotland. In this respect Northern Ireland is similar to England and Wales.

**General practice spotter
schemes**

3.69 There are no general practitioner spotter practices in Northern Ireland covering foodborne illness. **We recommend that consideration be given by DHSS(NI), in consultation with the Royal College of General Practitioners, to including some practices in Northern Ireland in the general practice spotter schemes existing or being developed in Great Britain** (R(II)3.14).

Sources of information on outbreaks

3.70 Although information on extensive outbreaks is reported to the DHSS(NI) so that the Department can co-ordinate investigation and control measures, there is no systematic recording of outbreaks by DHSS(NI). If necessary, the Department passes on information on outbreaks to the other Health Departments in the United Kingdom and to CDSC, Colindale. **We recommend that, wherever feasible, all outbreaks in the province are reported to DHSS(NI) and summaries and statistics published at least annually that are comparable with other foodborne outbreak data in the United Kingdom** (R(II)3.15).

Food Hazard warnings

3.71 Hazard warnings in relation to potential food poisoning risks are issued by DHSS(NI) to all Health Boards and District Council EHOs in the province.

Guidance on the management of outbreaks

3.72 In 1988 DHSS(NI) published guidance on the management of food poisoning and gastroenteritis in the community in a booklet entitled: "Memorandum on the Investigation and Control of Food Poisoning and Gastroenteritis in the Community". The Committee considers this booklet to be a helpful guide to the management of food poisoning outbreaks. However, we believe that there should be a consistency of approach between the countries of the UK in guidance provided on the management of outbreaks (see also paragraph 3.24).

Publication of information

3.73 Information on notifiable diseases, including food poisoning, is made available by DHSS(NI) in the monthly report "Communicable Diseases, Northern Ireland". This publication also contains information obtained from reports of laboratory isolations from humans, and from animals, forwarded to DHSS(NI) by the hospital laboratories and by the Veterinary Research Laboratory of DANI (see paragraph 3.86(b) below), respectively. As noted in paragraph 3.66 above, the Registrar General's Office of Northern Ireland also publishes quarterly and annual reports of notifiable diseases.

TRENDS IN FOODBORNE ILLNESS IN NORTHERN IRELAND

3.74 Statutory notifications of clinically diagnosed cases of food poisoning for the years 1975-1989 for Northern Ireland, Scotland and for England and Wales are set out in Table 3.1. The rates per 100,000 population are shown in Table 3.1 and Figure 3.2. The notification rates for Northern Ireland should be compared with formal notifications plus those ascertained by other means (see paragraph 3.67). As in other parts of the UK, the rate of food poisoning notified in Northern Ireland has increased since the mid 1980s; from 9.3 per 100,000 population in 1984 to 30.5 per 100,000 in 1989 with a fall in 1988 and a subsequent rise again in 1989. These rates are much lower than those reported for the same years in England and Wales (41.6 per 100,000 in 1984 and 103.8 per 100,000 in 1989). In England and Wales there was a pronounced increase in 1988 at the same time as a fall in Northern Ireland.

3.75 Trends in the laboratory reports to DHSS(NI) for gastrointestinal pathogens in the 1980's (Figure 3.1B) were similar to England and Wales except for salmonellas (see Part I, Figure 2.2). There was a peak of salmonellosis in Northern Ireland in 1987, which was accounted for, at least in part, by two outbreaks.

3.76 The changes in the total number and rates of salmonellas reported by microbiological laboratories in Northern Ireland (Table 3.2B, Figure 3.3) reflected the increase in notifications of food poisoning. Laboratory reports increased by about 50% during the 1980's compared with 130% in England and Wales. However, while the rates continued to increase in England and Wales in 1988 and 1989 (Table 3.2C), in Northern Ireland they fell in 1988 and remained constant in 1989 (Table 3.2B, Figure 3.3). This fall was in both *S. typhimurium* and *S. enteritidis* (Table 3.2B, Figure 3.4, 3.5).

3.77 During the early 1980s, while there was a slow increase in the rate of laboratory reports of *S. enteritidis* in England and Wales, the number of reports of

S. enteritidis in Northern Ireland remained very low until 1987 when there was a marked increase from 0.5 per 100,000 to 14.3 per 100,000, exceeding the rate in England and Wales for that year (Figure 3.5). However, while rates in England and Wales continued to increase in 1988 and levelled off in 1989, the rates fell in Northern Ireland after 1987.

3.78 In 1988 about 55% of the isolations of salmonella were identified as *S. enteritidis* most of which were phage type 4. The proportion of isolations of this serotype represents a marked increase from 1980 where isolations of *S. enteritidis* accounted for only 4% of the total. In Great Britain many of the cases of food poisoning over this period were associated with *S. enteritidis* and in a number of outbreaks in England and Wales the vehicle of infection has been identified as a product containing raw or undercooked eggs. In Northern Ireland no outbreaks of food poisoning have been detected in which eggs were the source of infection. Bacteriological examination of bulk raw eggs has been used to screen for the presence of *S. enteritidis* from 1988. None has been found, apart from one instance in 1989 when the source was traced to an infected flock which was subsequently slaughtered. In the circumstances no warning has been issued to the public about the consumption of raw eggs.

3.79 The number of reported isolations of campylobacter in Northern Ireland increased in the 1980s as in England and Wales and in Scotland (Table 3.3). However, the rates were very much lower than elsewhere in the UK (Figure 3.6).

3.80 Laboratory reports of listeriosis remained very low during the 1980s with between zero and two cases per year, apart from the increase in 1987, 1988 and 1989 (Table 3.4). This took place at about the same time as the increase occurred in the remainder of the UK.

Compatibility of data

3.81 The view expressed in paragraph 3.38 above on the need for a standardisation of data collection and reporting in the UK applies equally to Northern Ireland.

LABORATORY FUNDING AND ORGANISATION

3.82 As indicated in paragraph 3.61, there is no organisation in NI equivalent to the PHLS in England and Wales. The regional public health function is carried out in Northern Ireland at the Belfast City Hospital while microbiological investigations of local cases of food poisoning are carried out at hospital laboratories throughout the province. DHSS(NI) provides funding for regional services and within this allocation of funds the Eastern Health and Social Services Board allocates money to Belfast City Hospital for public health work generally. Additional money has recently been allocated to the Belfast City Hospital for extra consultant and scientific staff specifically to support the work on the investigation of foodborne illness including food surveillance. We welcome this development.

FOOD SURVEILLANCE

3.83 Responsibility for food surveillance and for the enforcement of the Food (NI) Order 1989 and Regulations lies with EHOs employed by District Councils. Bacteriological testing of samples taken locally, normally at the point of retail sale, is carried out at Belfast City Hospital. While District Councils receive reports on samples submitted locally there is no central collation of such data which could then be used to provide an overall analysis of the results of this testing programme in Northern Ireland. **We recommend that DHSS(NI) arrange for the central collation and analysis of the results of tests on food samples taken by environmental health officers in Northern Ireland** (R(II)3.16).

3.84 DANI is responsible for food surveillance in relation to milk on dairy farms and to liquid milk plants. In addition there is a specialist food microbiology centre which supports the DANI food control function and which has carried out surveys to detect particular organisms, such as Yersinia, Listeria, Staphylococcus, Salmonella and Campylobacter at processing plants. **We recommend that DHSS(NI) should collate the results of tests and surveys of food carried out by the Department of Agriculture for Northern Ireland together with those from the sampling programme undertaken by environmental health officers** (R(II)3.17).

ORGANISATION OF VETERINARY SERVICES IN NORTHERN IRELAND

3.85 Veterinary activities associated with the protection of public health are all located within DANI.

3.86 The Veterinary Division of DANI, headed by the Chief Veterinary Officer, performs the following functions:—

a. at local level, through ten geographic divisions each headed by a Divisional Veterinary Officer (DVO), it conducts on-farm investigation of zoonotic disease, routinely for brucellosis and tuberculosis, and for other diseases as necessary. The DVO liaises with the local Director of Public Health in relation to zoonotic diseases, providing the veterinary input into the area control of communicable disease team where necessary. Legal restrictions are applied where appropriate and advice is given to farmers and/or their veterinary practitioners on eradication of zoonotic diseases;

b. centrally, the Division receives statutory notifications regarding isolations of designated zoonotic organisms, and outbreaks of zoonotic diseases, in animals. It passes these to DHSS(NI), to the Director of Public Health of the appropriate Health Board, and to the Divisional Veterinary Officer for the area concerned when he is not himself the source of the notification. The information is also published by DHSS(NI) in its monthly report: "Communicable Diseases, Northern Ireland" — see paragraph 3.73, above. The Division also provides advice on any animal aspects of zoonotic disease, either directly to medical staff at DHSS(NI) or, where advice is needed locally, through the local DVO to the CCDC charged with control of communicable disease.

3.87 A Veterinary Research Laboratory is located within DANI. It is under the direction of the Chief Scientific Officer of DANI. This laboratory carries out most of the microbiological examination in Northern Ireland of samples from domesticated animals and birds and their environments. It is thus the main source of notifications reaching DANI's Veterinary Division as described at paragraph 3.86(b) above.

3.88 These veterinary activities are well integrated into the arrangements for making and operating policy on the control and prevention of foodborne illness in the province. Veterinary laboratory services, veterinary field services, and policy in relation to animal aspects of zoonoses, are all under the command of a single official, the Permanent Secretary, at DANI. Further, the senior staff involved in both DANI and DHSS(NI) are located in the same building and are in regular day-to-day contact. Coordination both within and between the two Departments appears to be highly effective.

COORDINATION BETWEEN THE DISCIPLINES INVOLVED

3.89 The control of communicable disease at sub-Regional or at Area Board Level is carried out by an Area Team led by the CCDC. It comprises a nurse, an EHO and, where necessary, a DVO of DANI. This team can call upon the RCDLG (see paragraph 3.59) for assistance at any time.

3.90 Monitoring and investigations may be triggered centrally by human infections, by animal infections or more rarely, by microbiological or chemical contamination of specific foods or food products. While the initial finding can be reported by any of the Departments mentioned above, the RCDLG provides the forum for coordinated action.

3.91 In general we found the arrangements for the monitoring and control of food poisoning to be well developed in Northern Ireland. Undoubtedly the situation is greatly helped by the relatively small size of the province when compared with England and Wales, or even with Scotland. In addition there are clearly advantages, which are not readily available elsewhere in the UK, that flow from having the key people in DANI and DHSS(NI) closely located in the same building.

Figure 3.1A
LABORATORY REPORTS OF GASTROINTESTINAL INFECTIONS
Scotland 1980-1989

Number of cases

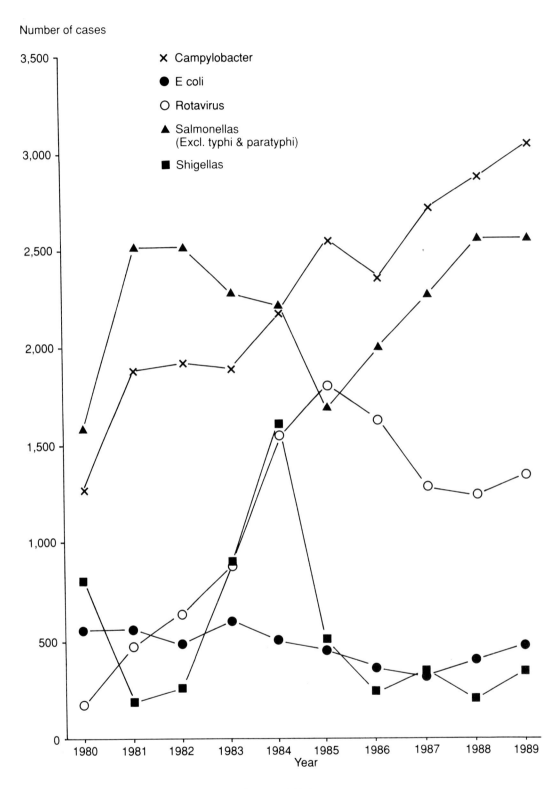

Source: Communicable Diseases (Scotland) Unit

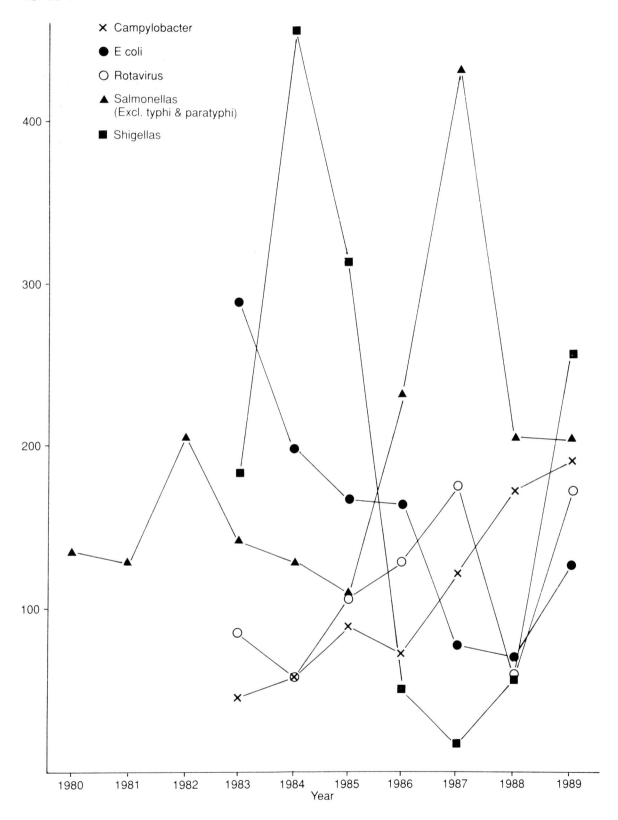

Figure 3.1B
LABORATORY REPORTS OF GASTROINTESTINAL INFECTIONS
Northern Ireland 1980-1989

Number of cases

× Campylobacter
● E coli
○ Rotavirus
▲ Salmonellas
  (Excl. typhi & paratyphi)
■ Shigellas

Year

Source: DHSS (NI)
Except for salmonellas. figures are not available pre-1983

41

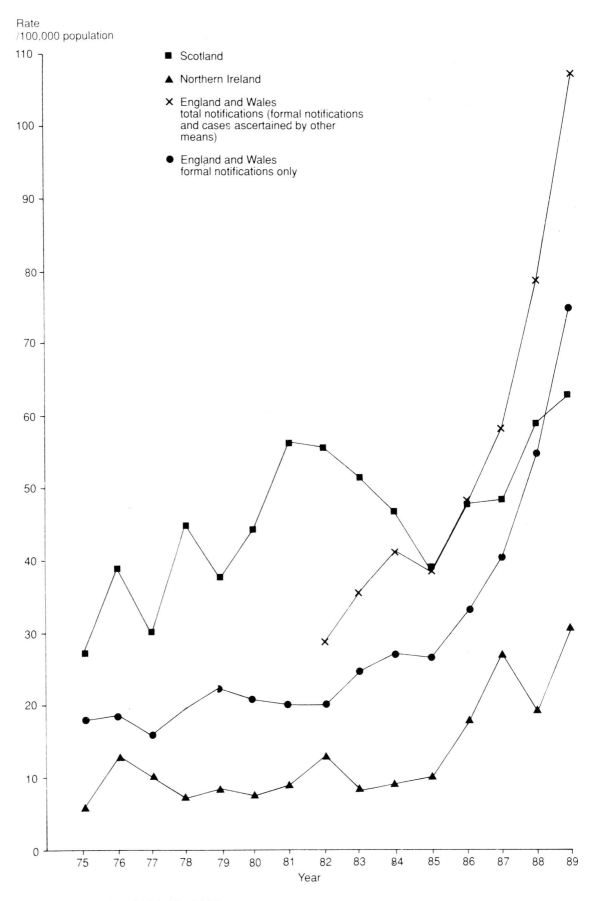

Figure 3.2
NOTIFICATIONS OF FOOD POISONING 1975-1989
Scotland, Northern Ireland and England and Wales

Rate
/100,000 population

■ Scotland

▲ Northern Ireland

✕ England and Wales
total notifications (formal notifications
and cases ascertained by other
means)

● England and Wales
formal notifications only

Year

Source: CD(S)U, DHSS (NI), OPCS

Figure 3.3
SALMONELLOSIS: LABORATORY REPORTS — ALL SALMONELLAS
Scotland, Northern Ireland and England and Wales

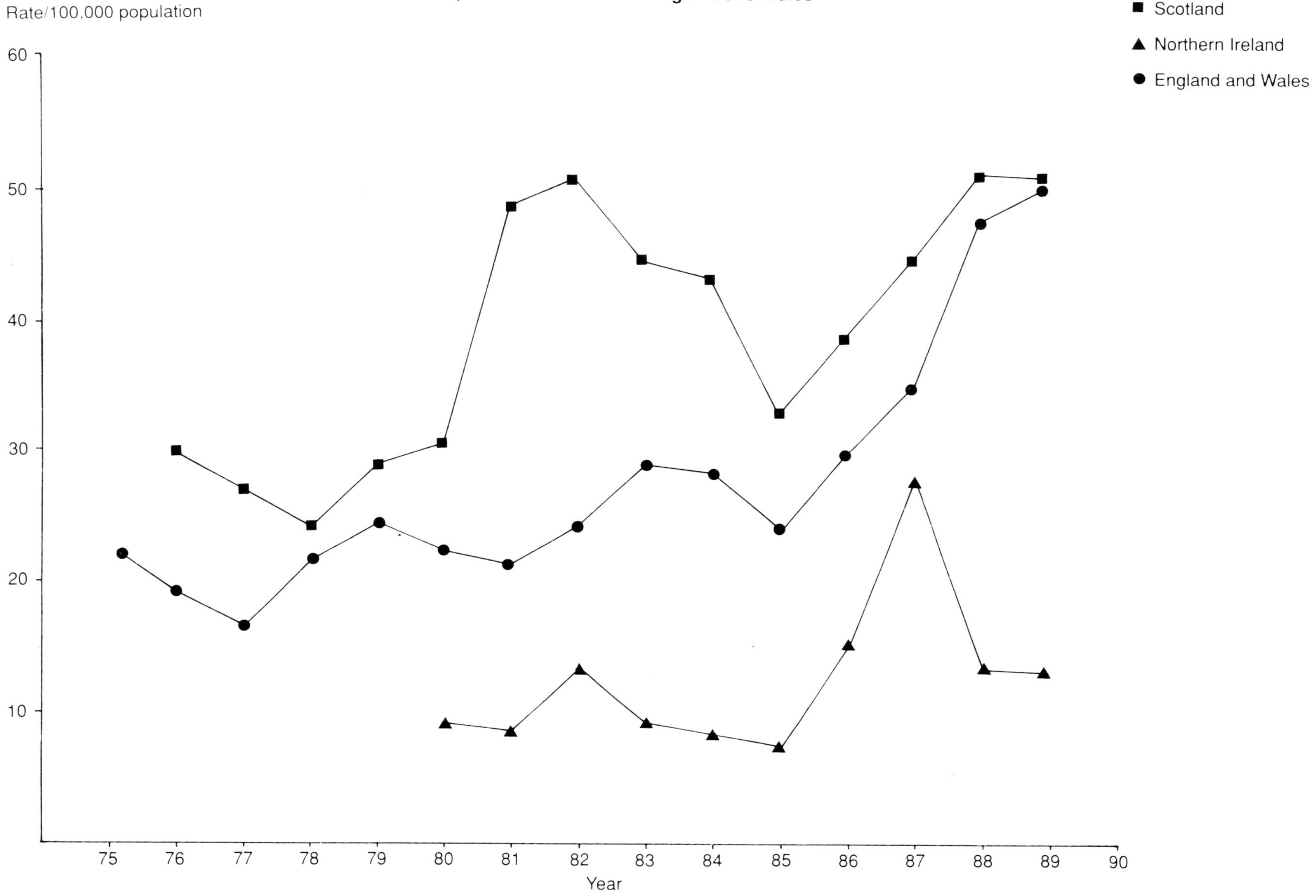

■ Scotland
▲ Northern Ireland
● England and Wales

Rate/100,000 population

Year

Source: CD(S)U. DHSS (NI), CDSC

43

Figure 3.4
SALMONELLOSIS: LABORATORY REPORTS — SALMONELLA TYPHIMURIUM
Scotland, Northern Ireland and England and Wales

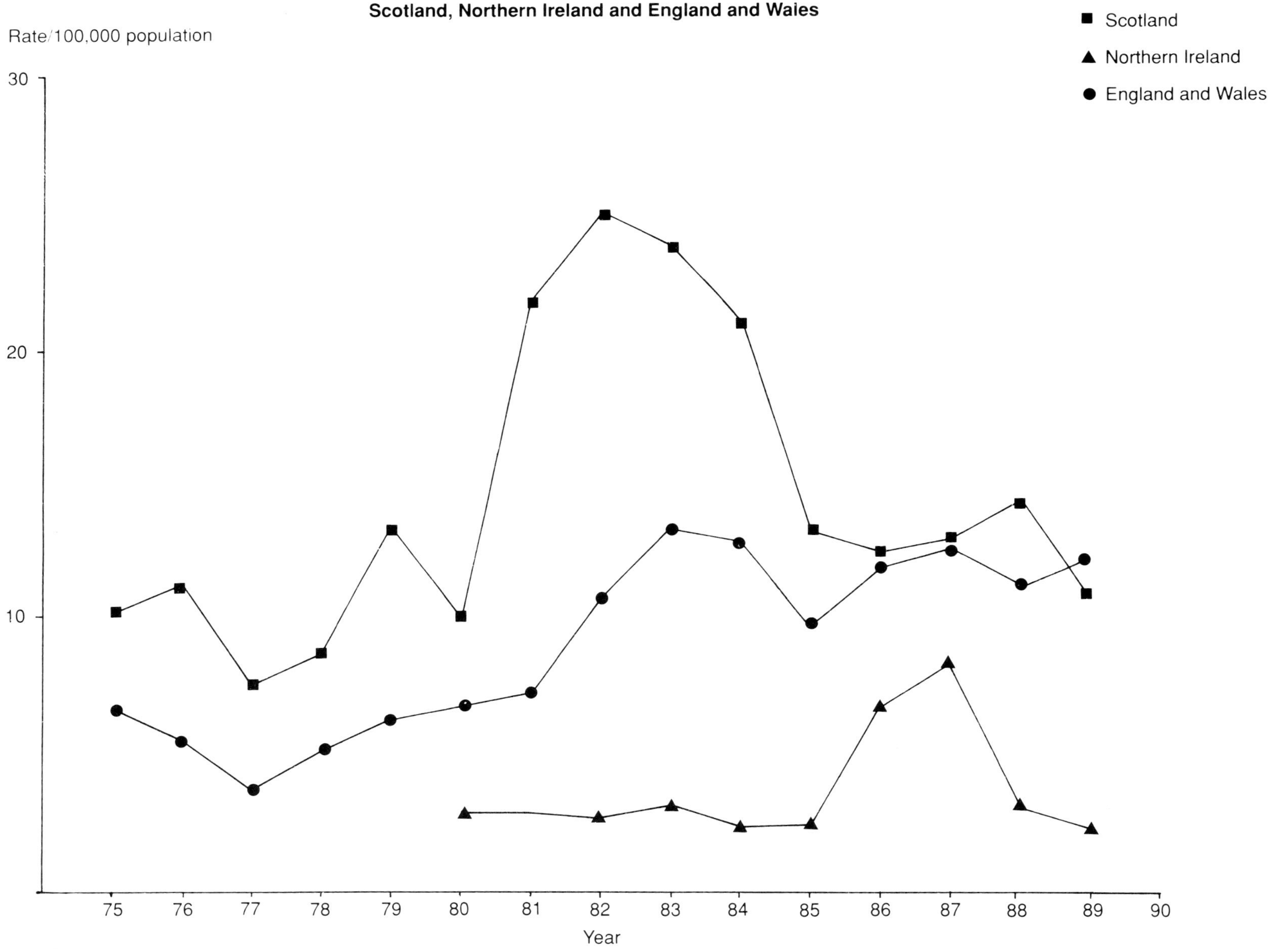

Rate/100,000 population

■ Scotland
▲ Northern Ireland
● England and Wales

Year

Source: CD(S)U, DHSS (NI), CDSC

44

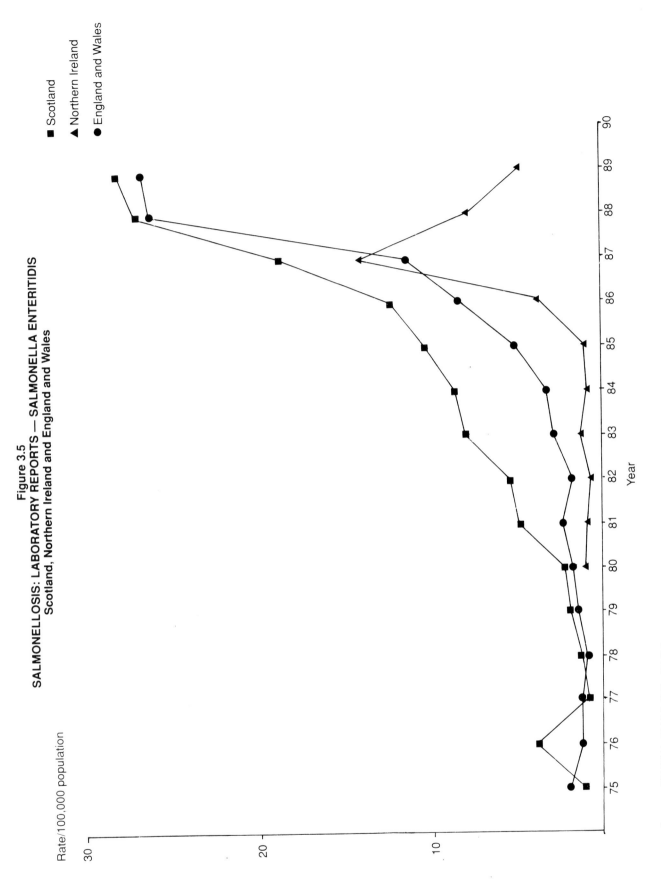

Figure 3.5
SALMONELLOSIS: LABORATORY REPORTS — SALMONELLA ENTERITIDIS
Scotland, Northern Ireland and England and Wales

■ Scotland
▲ Northern Ireland
● England and Wales

Rate/100,000 population

Year

Source: CD(S)U, DHSS (NI), CDSC

45

Figure 3.6
CAMPYLOBACTER: LABORATORY REPORTS
Scotland, Northern Ireland and England and Wales

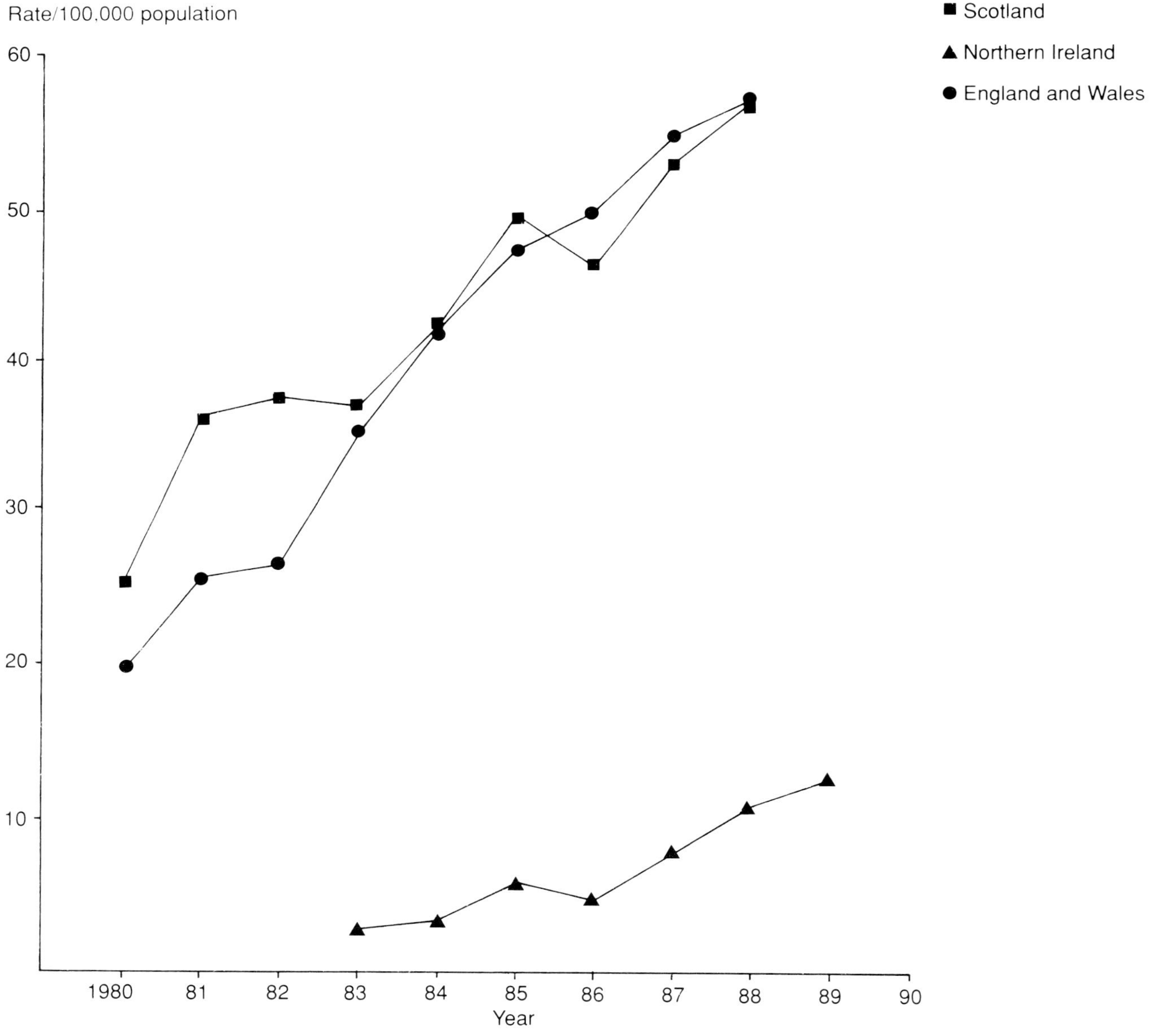

■ Scotland
▲ Northern Ireland
● England and Wales

Rate/100.000 population

Year

Source: CD(S)U, DHSS (NI), CDSC

46

Table 3.1 Food poisoning: Statutory Notifications
Scotland, Northern Ireland, England and Wales 1975-1989

	Scotland			Northern Ireland			England and Wales				
Year	Mid-year population in 1000's	Notifications	Rate/ 100,000 population	Mid-year population in 1000's	Notifications	Rate/ 100,000 population	Mid-year population in 1000's	Formal Notifications	Rate/ 100,000 population	Formal notifications + ascertained by other means	Rate/ 100,000 population
1975	5,206	1413	27.1	1,584	86	5.4	49,219	8,878	18.0		
1976	5,205	2023	38.9	1,524	202	13.3	49,154	9,226	18.8		
1977	5,196	1563	30.1	1,523	154	10.1	49,120	7,933	16.2		
1978	5,179	2319	44.8	1,523	109	7.2	49,117	9,741	19.8		
1979	5,167	1937	37.5	1,528	131	8.6	49,171	11,090	22.6		
1980	5,194	2299	44.3	1,533	114	7.4	49,603	10,318	20.8		
1981	5,167	2920	56.4	1,538	135	8.8	49,634	9,936	20.0		
1982	5,167	2880	55.7	1,538	198	12.9	49,601	9,964	20.1	14,253	28.0
1983	5,150	2632	51.5	1,543	128	8.3	49,654	12,273	24.7	17.735	35.7
1984	5.146	2391	46.5	1,551	144	9.3	49,764	13,247	26.6	20,702	41.6
1985	5,137	1967	38.3	1,558	158	10.1	49,924	13,143	26.3	19,242	38.5
1986	5,121	2436	47.6	1,567	273	17.4	50,075	16,502	33.0	23,948	47.8
1987	5,112	2480	48.5	1,575	423	26.9	50,243	20,363	40.5	29,331	58.4
1988	5,094	2998	58.9	1,578	302	19.1	50,393	27,826	55.2	39,713	78.8
1989	5,091	3204	62.9	1,583	483	30.5	50,562	38,042	75.2	52,492	103.8

1989 data provisional

Table 3.2 Salmonellosis : Laboratory reports of faecal isolates

Year	All salmonellas		S. typhimurium		S. enteritidis	
	No.	rate/ 100,000 population	No.	rate/ 100,000 population	No.	rate/ 100,000 population
A - SCOTLAND 1975-1989 – Reports to CD(S)U						
1975	1157	22.2	520	10.0	50	1.0
1976	1550	29.7	604	11.6	203	3.9
1977	889	17.1	392	7.5	24	0.5
1978	1253	24.2	455	8.8	68	1.3
1979	1483	28.7	700	13.5	84	1.6
1980	1577	30.4	522	10.1	113	2.2
1981	2526	48.8	1117	21.6	250	4.8
1982	2621	50.7	1286	24.9	279	5.4
1983	2288	44.4	1201	23.3	319	8.2
1984	2221	43.2	1069	20.8	433	8.4
1985	1690	32.9	689	13.4	528	10.3
1986	2015	39.3	649	12.6	619	12.1
1987	2286	44.7	679	13.3	940	18.4
1988	2580	50.6	737	14.5	1345	26.4
1989	2578	50.4	532	10.5	1402	27.5
B - NORTHERN IRELAND 1980-1989 – Reports to DHSS (NI)						
1980	136	8.9	44	2.9	6	0.4
1981	131	8.5	43	2.8	8	0.5
1982	207[1]	13.5	42	2.7	1	0.1
1983	141	9.1	49	3.2	12	0.8
1984	130	8.4	31	2.0	8	0.5
1985	115	7.4	36	2.3	8	0.5
1986	234	14.9	106	6.8	59	3.8
1987	433	27.5	133	8.4	225	14.3
1988	206	13.1	43	2.7	114	7.2
1989	205[2]	13.0	36	2.3	63	4.0
C - ENGLAND AND WALES 1975-1989 – Reports to CDSC						
1975	11271	22.6	3306	6.7	946	1.9
1976	9745	19.8	2962	6.0	586	1.2
1977	7998	16.3	1895	3.9	369	0.8
1978	10497	21.4	2650	5.4	737	1.5
1979	11940	24.3	3213	6.5	785	1.6
1980	10768	21.7	3513	7.1	816	1.6
1981	10539	21.2	3691	7.4	1110	2.2
1982	11987	24.1	5337	10.8	959	1.9
1983	14240	28.7	6741	13.6	1537	3.1
1984	14025	28.2	6369	12.8	1554	3.1
1985	11765	23.6	4780	9.6	2520	5.0
1986	14800	29.6	5885	11.8	4001	8.0
1987	17552	34.9	6400	12.7	5784	11.5
1988	23821	47.3	5566	11.0	13051	25.9
1989	24732	48.9	6074	12.0	13011	25.7

1. Includes 125 cases of S. *infantis*
2. Includes 23 cases of S. *braenderup*. The outbreak was associated with the consumption of coleslaw prepared by a person who was not feeling well at the time.

1989 data provisional

Table 3.3 **Campylobacter: Laboratory Reports of Faecal Isolates**
Scotland, Northern Ireland, England and Wales 1980-1989

	Scotland		Northern Ireland		England & Wales	
	No.	rate/ 100,000 population	No.	rate/ 100,000 population	No.	rate/ 100,000 population
1980	1,273	24.5	N/A	N/A	8,956	18.1
1981	1,887	36.4	N/A	N/A	12,168	24.5
1982	1,922	37.2	N/A	N/A	12,797	25.8
1983	1,895	36.7	45	2.9	17,278	34.8
1984	2,181	42.4	58	3.7	21,018	42.2
1985	2,563	49.9	90	5.8	23,572	47.2
1986	2,372	46.3	73	4.9	24,809	49.5
1987	2,740	53.6	122	7.7	27,310	54.3
1988	2,906	57.0	173	11.0	28,761	57.1
1989	3,080	60.5	192	12.1	32,526	64.3

N/A not available
1989 data provisional
These data are laboratory reports to CD(S)U in Scotland, to CDSC in England and Wales and to DHSS(NI).

Table 3.4 **Listeriosis: Laboratory Reports**
Scotland, Northern Ireland, England and Wales 1980-1989

	Scotland No.	Northern Ireland No.	England & Wales No.
1980	10	N/A	75
1981	7	N/A	86
1982	8	2	75
1983	16	0	115
1984	9	0	115
1985	14	0	149
1986	10	0	137
1987	36	5	254
1988	36	10	281
1989	29	6	244

N/A not available
1989 data provisional
From 1983 in England and Wales laboratory reports to CDSC were integrated with reference laboratory data (Division of Microbiological Reagents and Quality Control).

Table 3.5 **Foodborne disease in Scotland: 1980-1988**

	1980	1981	1982	1983	1984	1985	1986	1987	1988	Total 1980-88
Outbreaks										
Household	98	177	196	220	186	135	133	176	147	1,468
General	49	61	80	58	70	50	51	58	72	549
Total	147	238	276	278	256	185	184	234	219	2,017
Persons involved										
Household	235	374	495	606	529	380	361	453	411	3,844
General	1,070	1,703	1,605	1,037	988	1,105	626	1,372	1,235	10,741
Total	1,305	2,077	2,100	1,643	1,517	1,485	987	1,825	1,646	14,585
Deaths										
Household	3	2	1	3	—	1	1	—	—	11
General	3	11	1	3	1	4	3	2	2	30
Total	6	13	2	6	1	5	4	2	2	41

Source: CD(S)U

Table 3.6 **Outbreaks, number of persons involved and deaths — Scotland:**
by type of outbreak and aetiological agent: 1988
Number of persons hospitalised: by aetiological agent: 1988

	Aetiological Agent										
	Bacillus species	Campylo bacter	Clos perf	Salmo-nella	Salmon-Campylo	Shigella	Staphylo coccus	Viral Hepatitis	Other Toxins*	Un-known	Total
Houshold											
Outbreaks	2	18	1	114	1	1	1	—	2	7	147
Persons	9	52	2	309	5	4	5	—	7	18	411
Deaths	—	—	—	—	—	—	—	—	—	—	—
General											
Outbreaks	3	1	10	41	—	1	—	1	4	11	72
Persons	18	6	232	767	—	4	—	5	17	186	1,235
Deaths	—	—	—	2	—	—	—	—	—	—	2
Total Outbreaks	**5**	**19**	**11**	**155**	**1**	**2**	**1**	**1**	**6**	**18**	**219**
Total Persons	**27**	**58**	**234**	**1,076**	**5**	**8**	**5**	**5**	**24**	**204**	**1,646**
Total Hospitalised	**—**	**4**	**6**	**101**	**—**	**—**	**—**	**1**	**2**	**3**	**117**
Total Deaths	**—**	**—**	**—**	**2**	**—**	**—**	**—**	**—**	**—**	**—**	**2**

*Includes one outbreak where aetiological agent was chemical
Source: CD(S)U

Table 3.7 **Salmonellosis: Food Vehicles — Scotland**
General Community & Institutional Outbreaks reported to CD(S)U: 1986-1989

		Egg	Poultry	Others	Not Known	Total
1986 S.enteritidis	(PT4)	—	1(—)	—	2	3(—)
S.typhimurium		—	2	3	—	5
Other						
salmonellas		—	3	1	2	6
1987 S.enteritidis	(PT4)	1(1)	5(3)	1(1)	1(—)	8(5)
S.typhimurium		—	4	3	4	11
Other						
salmonellas		—	3	1	2	6
1988 S.enteritidis	(PT4)	4(3)	4(4)	2(2)	3(2)	13(11)
S.typhimurium		1	6	4	3	14
Other						
salmonellas		—	—	—	—	—
1989 S.enteritidis	(PT4)	4(4)	3(3)	—	3(3)	10(10)
S.typhimurium		—	1	3	2	6
Other						
salmonellas		—	1	3	2	6
TOTAL		**10**	**33**	**21**	**24**	**88**

Source: reports to CD(S)U from Scottish Salmonella Reference Laboratory, consultants in public health medicine and local authority environmental health departments.

ANNEX 3.1

SCOTLAND:
NOTIFIABLE INFECTIOUS DISEASES

Diseases notifiable by virtue of the 1988 Regulations

Anthrax
Bacillary Dysentery
Chickenpox
Food Poisoning
Legionellosis
Leptospirosis
Malaria
Measles
Meningococcal Infection
Mumps
Plague
Poliomyelitis
Rabies
Rubella
Tetanus
Tuberculosis
Viral Haemorrhagic Fevers
Viral Hepatitis
Whooping Cough

Diseases notifiable by virtue of the 1989 Regulations

Lyme Disease
Toxoplasmosis

Diseases notifiable by virtue of the 1988 Regulations and to which the Infectious
Disease (Notification) Act 1889 applies

Smallpox
Cholera
Diphtheria
Membranous Croup
Erysipelas
Scarlet Fever
Fevers known by any of the following names:— typhus, typhoid, enteric, relapsing,
continued or puerperal.

ANNEX 3.2

SCOTLAND:
REPORTABLE INFECTIONS
(as of 1st January 1990)

Actinomycosis
Amoebic infection (E. histolytica)
Atypical mycobacterial infection
Babesiosis
Bacterial Meningitis*
—*H. influenzae*
—*N. meningitidis*
—*S. pneumoniae*
Botulism
Brucellosis
Campylobacter (*C.jejuni*/*C.coli*) infection
Chlamydia psittaci
Clostridium difficile infection
Coxsackie infection (total)
Cryptosporidiosis
Cytomegalovirus
Echovirus infection (total)
E.coli 0157:H7 infection
Giardiasis
Human parvovirus infection
Hydatid disease
Leprosy
Listeriosis
Methicillin-resistant *S. aureus* infection
Q fever
Rotavirus infection
Salmonellosis
Tapeworm infection
Toxocariasis
Viral meningitis*
—Coxsackie
—Echovirus
—Mumps
Yersiniosis

*isolated from Cerebro Spinal Fever

ANNEX 3.3

SCOTLAND:
INFORMATION RECEIVED FROM
VETERINARY INVESTIGATION
SERVICE BY CD(S)U

The Veterinary Investigation Service reports to CD(S)U laboratory evidence of infections in animals or birds which are liable to cause illness in humans. Such reports would include:

Salmonellosis
Leptospirosis
Anthrax
Chlamydial infection
Listeriosis
Campylobacter infection
Q fever
Brucellosis
Toxoplasmosis

CHAPTER 4

RED MEAT PRODUCTION

INTRODUCTION

4.1 This chapter deals with the successive stages of red meat production. It first examines the background and the legal controls applied by both UK and EC legislation, and then undertakes a stage by stage examination of the production chain, seeking to identify the critical points in the rearing, transport and slaughter of livestock and the production of meat. A flow chart summarising the sector is at Figure 4.1. This is reproduced with the kind permission of the International Commission on Microbiological Specifications for Foods (ICMSF); it also portrays the ICMSF's assessment of the sources of contamination and critical control points in the red meat production chain, an assessment which coincides substantially with our own.

BACKGROUND

4.2 Red meat (beef, pork and lamb) is a major item in the national diet. In 1989 it accounted for an estimated 18% of household expenditure on food, with around £3 billion being spent on beef, £3 billion on pork and £1 billion on lamb. Output of red meat in 1989 was worth over £4 billion to UK farmers, representing 31% of their total output. Red meat accounted for 17% of food exports and 13% of food imports. There are 689 red meat slaughterhouses in England, 57 in Wales, 68 in Scotland and 22 in Northern Ireland, making a total of 836 in the UK.

4.3 As with poultry meat (see Part I, Chapter 6), there are no authoritative or systematic figures on the extent to which meat emerging from the slaughterhouse is contaminated with particular pathogenic microorganisms. However, a research project and a review carried out during the early 1980s by the Institute of Food Research of the Agricultural and Food Research Council (AFRC) gives some helpful indications. The research found that total viable surface bacterial counts of 10^3-10^4/cm^2 appeared to be very common, but that 10^2-10^3/cm^2 was achievable with care. It is clear that, in red meat, salmonella contamination is not as extensive as in poultry. The consensus of expert opinion seems to be that no more than 1% of beef and lamb carcases, though a higher percentage of pig carcases, carry salmonella when they enter chill. Other microorganisms that are, at least potentially, pathogenic to man have on occasion been isolated from red meat. These include *Clostridium perfringens, Listeria spp, Yersinia spp, Campylobacter spp, Staphylococcus aureus,* and *Escherichia coli.* The total number of microorganisms present in meat will tend to increase progressively following each subsequent handling stage.

4.4 We should stress that only in relation to some of these microorganisms has a link been demonstrated between their presence in red meat and foodborne illness; that the presence in red meat of low levels of bacteria which are in many cases widely present in the environment is not in itself cause for alarm; and that the problems that can arise from cross-contamination can be significantly minimised by the proper handling, storage and cooking of meat by all those involved, including the ultimate consumer.

4.5 The AFRC found that the incidence of bacteria in red meat was similar in seven EC countries which participated in a study. There is therefore no basis for

Figure 4.1
SOURCES OF CONTAMINATION AND CRITICAL CONTROL POINTS
BEFORE AND DURING SLAUGHTER OF RED MEAT ANIMALS

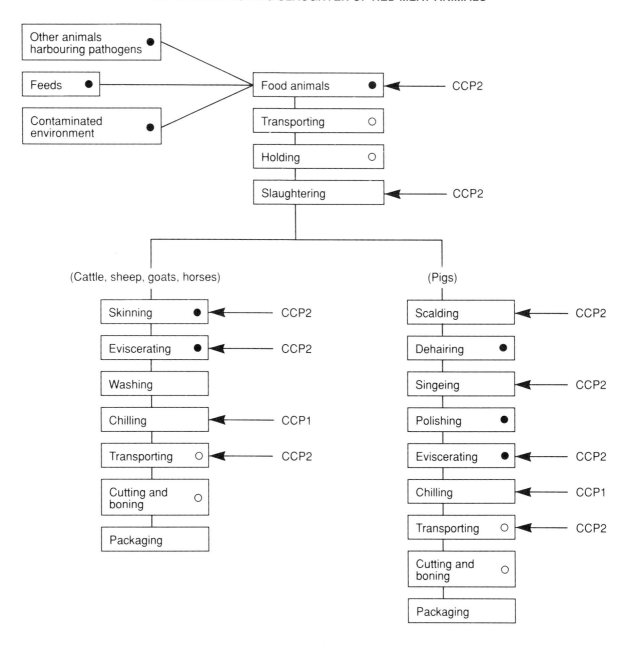

○ indicates a site of minor contamination

● indicates a site of major contamination

CCP1 effective CCP

CCP2 not absolute

Reproduced by kind permission of the International Commission on Microbiological Specifications for Foods

believing that the situation is different in the United Kingdom from that in other EC member states.

4.6 We are, however, firmly of the view that every effort must be made by all those involved in the initial stages of the red meat production chain to pass on a product in which microbiological contamination has been kept to the practical minimum. It is also vital that the working conditions — especially the speed of the line — should enable operatives to do their work with due care to minimise the risk of the carcase being contaminated.

LEGAL CONTROLS
General Animal Health Provisions

4.7 In Great Britain, the Zoonoses Order 1989 (which superseded an older version) designates salmonella and brucella organisms as a risk to human health. This designation is a procedure provided for in the Animal Health Act 1981, and enables various of the control powers in the Act to be used to deal with risks to human health as well as those to animal health. The Order requires the State Veterinary Service (SVS) to be notified when salmonella or brucella organisms are isolated from samples taken from, *inter alia*, farm animals and their carcases, products or surroundings. We have previously described (Part I, paragraph 6.13, first four indents) how the powers taken under the Order have been used to apply strict controls to the production of processed animal protein and animal feedingstuffs. In Northern Ireland, arrangements which are broadly similar to those described for Great Britain in this paragraph apply under the Zoonoses Order (Northern Ireland) 1976.

Provisions Relating to Slaughterhouses

4.8 In England and Wales, all slaughterhouses must be licensed by the local authority under the Slaughterhouses Act 1974. Licences are granted only to slaughterhouses that meet the requirements of secondary legislation made under the Slaughterhouses Act 1974 and the Food Act 1984. A comparable situation applies in Scotland, where "registration" of slaughterhouses by local authorities is conditional on compliance with the Slaughter of Animals (Scotland) Act 1956 and with relevant secondary legislation. Under the equivalent Northern Ireland arrangements, licensing is operated by the Department of Agriculture for Northern Ireland (DANI).

4.9 For slaughterhouses which supply the domestic market only, requirements on structure and hygiene are laid down in the Slaughterhouses (Hygiene) Regulations 1977, as amended, and in the Slaughterhouse Hygiene (Scotland) Regulations 1978, as amended. Enforcement is a local authority responsibility. The local authority also has a duty to provide a post mortem meat inspection service, as specified in the Meat Inspection Regulations 1987 and the Food (Meat Inspection) (Scotland) Regulations 1988. Inspection and the general supervision of standards is the responsibility of the local authorities (District Councils in England, Wales and Scotland), which are required to appoint Authorised Meat Inspectors (AMIs) to carry out the inspection duties. The AMIs normally work under the supervision of EHOs. Officers of the SVS visit plants annually to monitor standards and advise local authorities and plant operators on the standards to be met. In Scotland, the local authorities appoint Veterinary Meat Inspectors to judge and, if necessary, seize detained meat. Under the equivalent legislation in Northern Ireland, direct supervision of local authority slaughterhouses is the responsibility of the EHOs employed by the local authority, and other slaughterhouses are supervised by Government veterinarians.

4.10 Slaughterhouses approved for export to the EC are subject to additional requirements under the terms of EC Directive 64/433/EEC on intra-Community trade in fresh meat. These additional requirements are applied in England and Wales by the Fresh Meat Export (Hygiene and Inspection) Regulations 1987 and by equivalent legislation in Scotland and Northern Ireland. The requirements which apply in addition to those which must be met in order to supply the domestic market are briefly that:—

— additional structural requirements are applicable;

— veterinary ante mortem inspection is required. (However, this procedure is already routinely carried out in Scottish slaughterhouses which supply the domestic market. Also, Ministers announced in 1987 the Government's intention of introducing an ante mortem inspection requirement for production for the domestic market in England and Wales, in advance of the EC Commission's proposal (see paragraph 4.14 below) for an analogous requirement to be applied throughout the European Community);

— slaughterhouses must be approved to export to the EC by the appropriate Agriculture Minister in addition to being licensed/registered by the local authority;

— in addition to their general responsibility for day to day supervision, local authorities are required to appoint an Official Veterinary Surgeon (OVS), from a list compiled by the appropriate Agriculture Minister. The OVS takes overall responsibility for hygiene and inspection and applies the required export health marking;

— State Veterinary Service staff monitor standards in export-approved slaughterhouses on a monthly basis and advise local authorities and plant management on compliance with EC and UK requirements;

— EC Commission representatives periodically visit a sample of premises to assess compliance with Community requirements.

Ninety-six out of the 836 UK plants currently have approval for export to other EC member states — 54 out of 689 in England, three out of 57 in Wales, 24 out of 68 in Scotland and 15 out of 22 in Northern Ireland. Thus the majority of slaughterhouses in the United Kingdom supply the domestic market only. However, 43% of output comes from export-approved slaughterhouses.

4.11 Exports to countries outside the EC reflect the requirements of the importing countries concerned, and these arrangements remain under central Government control.

4.12 It should not automatically be supposed that those plants which do not have approval to export produce meat of a lower microbiological standard than export-approved ones. Many slaughter firms are content to supply the domestic market only, and so have no interest in obtaining approval to export. In any case the AFRC's work (see paragraph 4.3 above) showed that compliance with the structural requirements for export approval did not in itself result in the slaughterhouse concerned producing meat of high microbiological standard.

4.13 In England and Wales, meat deemed unfit for human consumption is subject to the Meat (Sterilisation and Staining) Regulations 1982 as amended. Equivalent legislation exists in Scotland and Northern Ireland. These regulations lay down requirements and restrictions — enforceable by local authorities — concerning the treatment and movement of unfit meat. They also prescribe the manner in which the parts of the carcase not intended for human consumption must be disposed of.

EC Proposals

4.14 The EC Commission's proposals to complete the Single Market (see Part II, paragraphs 1.25-1.28) envisage that, with the exception of ante mortem and certain other inspection provisions which would apply from 1 January 1991, the requirements which apply to export slaughterhouses would apply to all EC red meat plants from 1 January 1993.

4.15 It is envisaged by the EC Commission that some small operations might be granted exemption from the structural requirements detailed in the proposals, whilst others might be given temporary derogations to allow them time to bring themselves up to the required standards.

4.16 We welcome the fact that the Commission's proposals would lead to consistent requirements being applicable to all slaughterhouses within the European Community. We also welcome the fact that the proposed harmonised requirements envisage veterinary responsibility for hygiene and inspection matters, including ante mortem inspection: there are certain diseases which can be identified at ante mortem inspection, but which will show no pathological sign at post mortem inspection. We would deplore any derogations or exemptions from the control and inspection requirements.

4.17 The Commission's proposals have far-reaching implications for meat inspection arrangements. They could, for example, lead to the emergence of a larger cadre of professional veterinary meat hygiene specialists. We believe strongly that this should be the case. We believe that the need to implement new Community requirements will provide the Government with a valuable opportunity to appraise the current inspection arrangements in the United Kingdom and to make improvements. In particular, we consider the following aspects should be addressed:—

a. Staffing for meat inspection/meat hygiene enforcement arrangements. Following the rationalisation of the slaughtering industry which is expected to result from the stricter structural requirements, it may be that any shortage in the disciplines involved in inspection/enforcement will be substantially alleviated. However, it is clear that there will be a need for a greater number of suitably trained veterinary surgeons. It will also be necessary to ensure that the number of meat inspectors is adequate to meet the demands of modern higher-throughput plants.

b. The training of meat inspectors, veterinary surgeons and EHOs engaged in meat inspection. In our view a dedicated programme of training and continuing in-job development is required, in order to create an expert and committed cadre of staff.

c. The role of the OVS. OVSs may face a problem when meat hygiene considerations call for them to seek changes in the practices of the local authority which employs them. Regardless of the exact form of the future arrangements, we consider it important that the terms of OVSs' employment should not restrict their ability to make decisions as professionals.

d. The terms of employment of the OVS. Under current arrangements many OVSs are only employed by local authorities on one-year contracts, sometimes subject to competitive tendering. This militates against the development of a dedicated force of veterinary staff. The likely increase in the demand for OVSs makes it all the more important that they should be employed on a longer term basis.

e. Overall supervision of the meat inspection system. We feel there is a need for responsibility to be clearly allocated for overseeing the meat inspection system and ensuring high and consistent standards. In our view this responsibility should be given to the SVS.

4.18 **We recommend, once the new EC arrangements for meat inspection are agreed and ready for implementation:—**

i. **that the Government should ensure that provision is made**

— **for the training of a sufficient number of meat inspectors, Environmental Health Officers and veterinarians; and**

— **for the setting up of arrangements under which the disciplines involved act as a team led by the veterinary surgeon authorised for the purpose;**

ii. **that the appointment of the veterinary surgeon within the system should be on a longer term and a more permanent basis; and**

iii. **that the State Veterinary Service should be given explicit responsibility for overseeing the meat inspection and hygiene arrangements** (R(II)4.1).

STAGE-BY-STAGE CONSIDERATION OF THE PRODUCTION CHAIN

Rearing of Livestock

4.19 Action on the farm to minimise eventual contamination of red meat with pathogenic microorganisms should, in particular, anticipate the routes by which meat can potentially be contaminated. For example, microorganisms present in an animal's gastrointestinal tract may eventually contaminate the meat if the tract is handled unsatisfactorily during the dressing and evisceration process. Faecal contamination of an animal's coat or skin may result in the meat becoming soiled during the dressing process and contamination with any bacteria which may be present in the faeces. Apart from the hygiene implications, there are clearly good economic reasons for the industry to improve the cleanliness of animals presented for slaughter, since it has been estimated by representatives of the hide trade that the loss of income because of excessive soiling of hides is £20 million per annum. Again, if animals are in an unduly stressed condition at slaughter, this can result in their excreting microorganisms and contaminating other animals and the slaughterhouse environment. Farmers can therefore contribute to food safety by producing healthy, clean and unstressed animals for slaughter, and we believe that this simple truth should be constantly borne in mind by livestock producers and stressed by all who provide them with advice. Compliance with the codes of practice concerned with animal welfare and with farm building design, etc (see Annex 4.1) will contribute considerably in this context. We also consider that the reduction which is foreseen in the over-capacity in the slaughtering industry should create a more favourable climate than has hitherto existed for slaughterers to offer farmers a price structure which encourages the production of clean animals. **We recommend that abattoir managers should pay farmers a premium to take account of the cleanliness of the animals as one of the components of quality** (R(II)4.2).

4.20 Animal feedingstuffs have been shown to be a route by which pathogens such as salmonella are introduced into the food chain. The comments we made on feedingstuffs in our chapter on poultry meat (Part I, paragraphs 6.23-6.27) apply equally in the context of red meat production.

4.21 We previously noted (Part I, Appendix 3, paragraph A.3.5) that poorly-produced silage has been shown to be a source of listeriosis in ruminants, especially sheep and goats. Cattle are relatively resistant to listeriosis. Although sheep and goats are more susceptible, they present with an apparent encephalitis or an abortion accompanied by bacteraemia, and so are easily identified and not slaughtered for human consumption. It does not appear, therefore, that livestock sick with listeriosis are likely to be an important source of listeria in meat. Nor is there a significant degree of risk of meat becoming contaminated with *L. monocytogenes* through animals, without overt clinical signs, carrying the bacterium; careful handling of the gastrointestinal tract in the slaughterhouse will minimise any possibility of contamination.

4.22 A guiding principle for farmers in relation to intensive husbandry systems is that batches of animals should be handled on an "all in/all out" basis, with thorough and effective cleansing and disinfection in between. Buildings should also be designed, constructed, cleaned and managed in a way which as far as possible minimises access by birds, rodents and insects.

4.23 In extensive (as opposed to intensive) systems, there are clearly no effective control measures which can be applied against environmental contamination, eg from infected wild birds. However the provision of piped potable water, exclusion of access by animals to contaminated supplies, and local observation of proper precautions on the disposal of sewage sludge, effluent and farm slurry are all important.

4.24 Our comments on the rearing of livestock have all been made in relation to the rearing of animals specifically for meat production. More care may be required with other animals not primarily reared for human consumption such as cull cows, cull ewes and 'spent' bulls; such animals, because of their age or because they are being disposed of following health problems, are more likely to be carrying infections which would make them unfit for human consumption. We consider that the forthcoming introduction of ante mortem inspection is particularly welcome in relation to such animals. **We recommend that those carrying out ante mortem inspection should devote particular attention to cull animals** (R(II)4.3).

4.25 We consider that health records kept on the farm may potentially be of use to those who inspect meat in slaughterhouses. Hitherto it has not normally been practicable for inspectors to identify the farm of origin sufficiently quickly for this approach to be assessed (for example because animals may have passed through many hands between the farm of origin and the slaughterhouse). However electronic tagging is becoming feasible and is being introduced by some farmers. It might make on-farm health records more accessible, and enhance animal disease control by making information on animal movements much more comprehensive and accessible. We also consider that meat inspection is an area where electronic tagging will in the long term bring benefits — for example by enabling an inspector to have prompt access to animals' health records, and by facilitating the transmission of post mortem data back to the farmers. Its use for statutory purposes might pose problems, but we are aware of the technical progress that has been made in other countries. **We recommend that the Government should encourage technical developments in electronic tagging, and should be alert to any opportunity to put the practice to use in the control of animal disease** (R(II)4.4).

Transport and Marketing of Livestock

4.26 It is inevitable that animals will have to be transported to the abattoir, possibly via sale at auction and via dealers. Ideally this would not lead to increased faecal contamination of the coat or fleece, but in practice the mixing of animals with others in unfamiliar surroundings, possibly on several journeys, will increase stress leading to a greater faecal load and a higher risk of cross-contamination. As with on-farm husbandry, the principles for minimising stress on animals in transport and at market are well known, will help to reduce the number of microorganisms being introduced into the abattoir, and are embodied in the legislation and codes of practice relating to animal welfare. It is important that the industry should make the welfare of the animals a high priority at all times during transport and at market, and we urge local authorities to give a high priority to enforcing the relevant animal welfare legislation.

4.27 Young calves are susceptible to various ailments including salmonellosis. However, they are normally slaughtered at an age when they have recovered from such infections, which therefore do not in themselves present a significant food safety problem. Nonetheless, a reduction in the number of calves in transit would assist the production of microbiologically satisfactory meat by minimising the number of animals excreting salmonella and other organisms into lorries and the environment. We endorse the efforts that have been made by the British Veterinary Association and the Livestock Auctioneers Market Committee to reduce, through guidance, the repeated passage of young calves through livestock markets. We also welcome the fact that MAFF has issued proposals to introduce statutory requirements to prevent the practice.

4.28 Effective cleansing and disinfection of vehicles in between loads is statutorily required by the Transit of Animals (Road and Rail) Order 1975. The purpose is to prevent the spread of animal disease, but this should also contribute to the minimisation of microbial contamination in the slaughterhouse. It is apparent that the degree of enforcement of these regulations varies between local authorities. Some authorities operate a system whereby the driver is issued, on unloading at the livestock market or the abattoir, with a document which must subsequently be endorsed at the approved wash bay to show that cleansing and disinfection has been carried out. The haulier is not allowed to load further animals unless he has an endorsed document. We commend this system of documentation to local authorities as one effective way of enforcing the cleansing and disinfection requirements for lorries. To enable cleansing and disinfection to be carried out more easily, the approved washing facilities should be sited as near as possible to the market or abattoir. **We recommend that all new markets and abattoirs should have wash bay facilities for lorries on site or immediately adjacent** (R(II)4.5).

Slaughter

4.29 The following paragraphs examine those parts of the slaughter process that are of particular relevance in relation to microbiological contamination.

4.30 The lairage. The conditions of an animal's stay in the slaughterhouse lairage should minimise stress and thereby reduce faecal contamination. The relevant legislation (The Slaughter of Animals (Humane Conditions) Regulations 1990) lays down the requirements for the design of lairages. We stress the importance of:—

— the calm and unhurried droving of animals;

— good construction and design, with flooring in particular being of a suitable type and standard, and capable of being effectively cleansed and disinfected;

— the provision of facilities for isolation and veterinary clinical examination;

— cleansing and disinfection of the lairage between consignments;

— the provision of adequate and clean bedding where appropriate;

— in the case of pigs, spraying with water before stunning provided that ambient temperature and humidity are low, in order to reduce faecal contamination;

— the clipping of cattle and sheep along the intended lie of the incision for removal of the hide or fleece (see paragraph 4.33 below).

4.31 We believe that there is a risk attached to the practice of very young calves being kept in the lairage until sufficient numbers have been accumulated to justify economic slaughter. We understand that animals may legally be kept on the slaughterhouse premises for up to 72 hours before being slaughtered. However, if young calves are kept for more than a short time, any that are carrying salmonella organisms are highly likely to start excreting them, and quickly to infect other animals. It is highly undesirable to create a situation in which batches of calves are gathered which will excrete salmonella organisms into the slaughterhouse environment in this way. **We firmly recommend that all calves should be slaughtered on the day of arrival at the slaughterhouse** (R (II)4.6).

4.32 Stunning/bleeding. The first stages in the slaughter process involve the stunning of the animal, the hoisting of the animal by its hind legs on to the bleeding rail, and the severing of the main blood vessels in the neck. There is a risk with these procedures of microbiological contamination entering the animal from its skin via the implements used, or on occasions when inadvertently there is simultaneous severance of the blood vessels and oesophagus. **We recommend that a freshly sanitised knife be used for bleeding each animal** (R(II)4.7). Where pithing (physical destruction of brain tissue and spinal cord with a flexible rod inserted in the bolt hole at the front of the skull) is carried out in conjunction with captive bolt stunning to control post-stunning convulsions, this presents a significant microbiological risk, since blood is still pumping round the carcase and can carry to all parts of the body any microorganisms introduced. We consider that the use of modern stunning equipment and techniques removes the need for pithing, which might otherwise be necessary for the safety of the slaughterhouse operatives. **We recommend that the Government consider whether the practice of pithing should cease, as it introduces an unnecessary risk of contamination even if a sterilised pithing rod is used** (R(II)4.8).

4.33 Removal of hide/fleece (cattle/sheep). This is a critical point, since contact between the outer surface and the carcase is a prime source of faecal contamination. Care must be taken to avoid such contact, and to remove the hide or fleece promptly from the slaughter hall. The mechanised pulling systems now in general use represent a significant improvement over the traditional manual ones. The risk of contamination is particularly high with the traditional method of removing fleece from sheep as this involves a high degree of contact between the operators' hands, the fleece and the carcase. Apart from the practice of clipping the fleece along the intended line of incision (see paragraph 4.30 above), **we recommend the use of the new "inverted dressing" system for sheep which provides a much cleaner method of removing the fleece** (R(II)4.9).

4.34 Scalding/dehairing (pigs). Pigs are not commonly skinned, and so the reduction of faecal contamination on the carcase involves somewhat different considerations. The passage of the animals through a scald tank to facilitate the dehairing process is a hazard point. The water quickly accumulates microorganisms, and it is important to change it frequently, as well as to maintain it at a temperature of 62-65°C. Another risk is that inhalation can occur as a reflex action if pigs enter the scald tank less than six minutes after exsanguination. Contamination can also occur through water entering by the exsanguination cut. **Therefore we recommend to slaughterhouse managers that care must be taken to wait at least six minutes after bleeding before passing the pigs into the scald tank, that the temperature of the water should be monitored closely, and that the water should be frequently changed** (R(II)4.10). We found the singeing of the dehaired carcase, as carried out in some slaughterhouses, to be a desirable practice which is capable of eliminating most surface contamination. However, it is important that the washing and/or scrubbing which is subsequently carried out to remove carbon deposits does not result in recontamination of the carcase surface. The machine generally used for this process appears to be basically uncleanable. **We recommend that attention be paid to the hygienic aspects of the design of the machinery used for washing or scrubbing pig carcases** (R(II)4.11).

4.35 Freeing of the rectum/anus. The freeing of the anus from the surrounding tissue, and dropping of it into the abdominal cavity, is a practice that can cause faecal contamination through spillage of intestinal contents. Tying off the anus before dropping it into the cavity will reduce this risk. Work in Denmark with pigs has suggested that this problem can be reduced further if "tying and bagging" is carried out by enclosing the anus in a polythene bag with a rubber band round it. **We recommend that industry adopt the practice of tying and bagging, particularly for cattle and pigs, as soon as possible** (R(II)4.12).

4.36 A similar problem exists at the other end of the tract where the neck and head area can be contaminated with the contents of the rumen. To deal with this **we recommend that the oesophagus is sealed at the entrance to the rumen, which in cattle requires a rodding technique to be used. We also recommend that new plant should be designed to permit the use of the techniques necessary to achieve this** (R(II)4.13).

4.37 Evisceration. Rupture of the gastrointestinal tract and spillage of its contents is a prime source of microbial contamination. The points of greatest hazard are the cutting of the brisket and lifting out of the tract, in particular when the oesophagus and stomach are separated. Evisceration is therefore a major hazard point. There should be greater awareness of the risks because, given adequate time and proper supervision and care, removal of the tract to the gut room can be achieved without problem.

4.38 Plant and equipment. Much of the equipment involved in the slaughter process has been designed with speed of operation rather than hygiene as a priority. It is of vital importance that equipment in slaughterhouses and cutting plants, which comes into repeated contact with meat (eg transport belts, working surfaces, saws, etc) should be regularly and effectively cleansed and disinfected. **We recommend that in future those designing slaughter equipment should make ease of cleaning a high priority, and that management should make sure that staff are trained in the cleansing and disinfection procedures** (R(II)4.14).

4.39 Post mortem inspection. Historically, post mortem inspection was based on examination for tuberculosis, but the current meat inspection regulations reflect the changing disease pattern in livestock. Inspection focuses essentially on pathological lesions, and picks up post mortem conditions and cross-contamination, so that meat or offal can then be trimmed or condemned and disposed of under the Sterilisation and Staining Regulations (see paragraph 4.13 above).

4.40 Cleaning of carcases. With good hygiene and slaughter, dressing and evisceration practice, the carcase produced will in most cases not need washing. Should washing be needed, the volume of water must be kept to a minimum, and if possible must be carried out in a cabinet to minimise aerosol spread. Work has established the appropriate type of nozzle to produce a fine jet spray, and information on this can be found in Meat and Livestock Commission technical bulletins.

4.41 Chilling. Air chilling is the method used. To meet EC requirements, fresh meat for intra-Community trade must, by law, be chilled immediately after post mortem inspection, and be kept at a continuous internal temperature of not more than 7°C for carcase meat and 3°C for offal. There is provision for derogations to be granted to allow the warm cutting of bovine, sheep and pig carcases provided that the prescribed temperatures are reached within 48 hours (bovine) and 20 hours (sheep and pigs); several member states, including the UK, have been granted such derogations. Under the UK legislation which applies to "domestic" slaughterhouses, meat held in a slaughterhouse for 48 hours or more must be placed in refrigerated accommodation. The EC Commission's proposals for the Single Market would extend the requirements for "export" slaughterhouses to all slaughterhouses in the European Community.

4.42 In order to control microbial growth, chilling to below 7°C should take place as rapidly as possible, subject to the constraint that excessively fast chilling can lead to toughening of the meat. We therefore welcome the EC Commission's proposals to this effect, and the Government's support for them.

4.43 It is important that the installation of higher-speed and higher-capacity slaughter lines in slaughterhouses should be matched by the provision of chilling capacity sufficient to accommodate the throughput. If this is not the case cross-contamination will occur through contact between carcases or through the chilling process working slower than it should. Further, the fans used in air chilling can disseminate moulds and bacteria. It is therefore essential that chillers should be properly constructed and maintained. Design of chillers should be such as to provide for effective cleansing and disinfection, and for adequate circulation of air. Overcrowding with carcases must be avoided: poor air flow or contact between carcases will lead to cross-contamination and uneven chilling. **We recommend that particular attention be given to ensuring sufficient airflow and minimum contact between carcases in chill rooms** (R(II)4.15).

4.44 Speed of Working. A recurring theme of our analysis has been that in many different ways the high line speeds of modern abattoir equipment lead to increased microbiological hazard. This occurs, for example, when operations, such as removal of the hide or fleece or evisceration, have to be carried out at unduly high speed so that operatives cannot clean their hands and their implements between carcases. It also occurs because ease of cleaning and disinfection has not been given priority in the design of machinery intended to work at high speed. Another factor which encourages hasty working in abattoirs is the fact that workers are generally paid piece-rates. The research undertaken by the AFRC suggested that the skill and care exercised by slaughter/dressing operatives was of paramount importance to the production of a microbiologically satisfactory product. **We recommend that the industry ensures that all managers and operatives are aware of the importance of minimising contamination and the steps that should be taken to achieve this. We also recommend that enforcement officers should pay close attention to the hygiene implications of line speed when performing their duties and should not hesitate to insist on operations being suspended if practices are not satisfactory** (R(II)4.16).

4.45 Microbiological monitoring. We stress the important contribution that can be made by microbiological monitoring as an adjunct to the Hazard Analysis and Critical Control Point approach which we commend for the slaughterhouse as for all other stages of food production. Its regular application to key equipment and to the carcase at critical points in the process will determine 'normal' microbial levels in a given plant, and thus provide a valuable early indication when there is a breakdown in hygiene arrangements which needs attention. Monitoring should also be used to check the effectiveness of cleansing and disinfection. For this to be done effectively there is a need for a basis of equivalent methodology to be agreed. We consider that it would be highly desirable to extend and build on the AFRC's work (which was suspended five years ago) so as to determine the value of microbiological monitoring and the best methods of carrying it out. **We recommend the Steering Group on the Microbiological Safety of Food to consider how arrangements can best be made for the work formerly done by the Agriculture and Food Research Council on microbiological monitoring to be taken forward (R(II)4.17).**

BUTCHERY

4.46 After the animal has been slaughtered, dressed and chilled, the resulting carcase or part-carcase (e.g. beef quarter) is subjected to further treatment before the meat is used. Butchery subdivides the carcase or part-carcase into smaller portions, joints, cuts, etc. Simple processing including packaging may follow. Also, a significant amount of red meat is used in a wide variety of manufacturing processes, the microbiological safety implications of which we have already considered (Part I, Chapter 7).

4.47 Butchery can take place in premises adjacent to the slaughterhouse. Alternatively carcases can be transported to a large centralised butchery operation or to catering or retailing premises, either directly from the slaughterhouse or via a meat market.

4.48 The butchery of meat for the UK market only must conform to The Food Hygiene (General) Regulations 1970 and their equivalents in Scotland and Northern Ireland. Cutting plants may be approved for intra-Community trade in accordance with the Fresh Meat (Hygiene Inspection) Regulations 1987, which implement EC requirements.

4.49 As with slaughter and dressing, high standards of hygiene can be achieved in butchery if all concerned are aware of the microbiological risks and the steps necessary to minimise them. Operators must be adequately trained and well supervised.

Packaging

4.50 At some intermediate stage during butchery, primal cuts may be packaged, (eg vacuum packaged) for storage and/or distribution prior to final butchery, when the portions of meat may be pre-packed for retail sale. Such pre-packaging ranges in complexity from simple over-wrapping to packaging in material impermeable to gases and modifying the gaseous atmosphere in the pack, ie changing the concentrations of oxygen, nitrogen and carbon dioxide. Modified atmosphere packaging can help to maintain the colour of meat and to delay spoilage. While it is important that it is carried out hygienically and with good temperature control of the packaged product, there is no evidence that it presents any risks to health.

Minced Meat

4.51 A significant amount of meat (for example, approximately 25% of beef) is converted into minced meat which is used in catering and the home for a variety of cooked dishes and in manufacture of products ranging from burgers and sausages to canned products and chilled or frozen ready meals. While some minced meat is prepared from trimmings from the preparation of joints and cuts, much minced meat is prepared from parts of the carcase for which there is insufficient consumer demand as joints or cuts, e.g. fore-quarter beef or lamb breasts.

4.52 Minced meat spoils more rapidly than joints or cuts and therefore needs to be produced, and where necessary held, under strict temperature control. As with other forms of red meat, adequate training and supervision of operators is essential to minimise microbiological risks.

4.53 Our attention has been drawn to a draft EC Regulation laying down hygiene requirements for the production and placing on the market of minced meat. The purpose of the proposal is to harmonise rules for the sale of mince in the Single Market; however, we understand that the proposed rules take account of the fact that minced meat is sometimes consumed raw in some member states, and in so doing set requirements which are in our view unnecessarily restrictive for minced meat which is to be cooked before consumption. We note that the Regulation does not apply to minced meat prepared in and obtained from retail shops and which is unpackaged. Notwithstanding our observations in paragraph 4.52 above, we nevertheless consider that the proposed requirements are unnecessarily stringent in relation to minced meat produced in and for consumption in the UK, where minced meat is not normally consumed raw.

Mechanically Recovered Meat

4.54 Conventional methods of removing meat from bones during butchery leave a substantial quantity of meat adhering to the bone. This meat can be recovered by various kinds of machines. Such mechanically recovered meat is similar to conventional finely minced meat, conforms to the legal definition of meat, and is extensively used in manufactured meat products.

4.55 The bones from which mechanically recovered meat is produced must be handled as a source of food and not as waste material. High standards of hygiene and strict temperature controls must be applied both to the bones and to the mechanically recovered meat during its production and subsequent use. The British Meat Manufacturers' Association has produced a particularly useful Code of Practice for the preparation of mechanically recovered meat which we endorse. We are satisfied that mechanically recovered meat, if properly prepared, need not present a significant risk to public health from the microbiological point of view.

CONCLUSIONS

4.56 To a very substantial degree, the theme of this chapter is that high standards of hygiene can be achieved in red meat production if all concerned are fully aware of the microbiological risks and the steps that can be taken to minimise them. This applies to all stages from the farm to the cutting plant, and at many levels — from slaughterhouse workers being aware of the basic principles of personal hygiene to the design and selection of equipment.

ANNEX 4.1

LIST OF RELEVANT
CODES OF PRACTICE

a. ON ANIMAL WELFARE

i. On-farm

Codes of recommendations for the welfare of livestock:—

> Cattle
> Domestic Fowls
> Ducks
> Farmed Deer
> Goats
> Pigs
> Rabbits
> Sheep
> Turkeys

ii. In transit

Guidelines for the transport of farmed deer.

Code of practice on the care of farm animals and horses during their transport on roll-on/roll-off ferries.

Code of practice for the care and feeding of farm animals in government approved export lairages.

Code of practice for the transport by air of cattle, sheep, pigs, goats and horses.

Livestock shipments on Roll-on/Roll-off (Ro-Ro) vessels — Advice to Masters, Loading Officers and vessel operators.

b. ON BUILDING DESIGN

The British Standards Code of Practice for the Design of Buildings and Structures for Agriculture (BS 5502).

CHAPTER 5

MILK AND MILK PRODUCTS

INTRODUCTION

5.1 This chapter considers the dairy sector, which we have taken to comprise the production, processing and distribution of milk, and the manufacture of various milk products. The subject-area is thus diverse and is expanding with the development of various novel products. Figure 5.1 provides a diagram of the sector, and indicates the major regulatory controls already in place which have a bearing on health and hygiene. Technical detail, statistics and flow charts are included in appendices to the chapter. The chapter covers the following key areas:—

— a description of the sector, which puts it in perspective and gives some essential economic background (paragraphs 5.2-5.7);

— a review of the incidence of foodborne illness which has been associated with milk and milk products (paragraph 5.8);

— relevant legal measures, domestic and EC, present and proposed (paragraphs 5.9-5.19);

— consideration of the hygienic quality of milk marketed in the UK (paragraphs 5.20 and 5.21);

— a review, with recommendations where appropriate, of the critical points in the production and processing chain for

— liquid milk (paragraphs 5.22-5.36);

— cheese (paragraphs 5.37-5.52);

— other milk products (milk powders, yoghurt, ice cream, butter, and novel and composite milk products) (paragraphs 5.53-5.62).

THE DAIRY SECTOR IN PERSPECTIVE

5.2 The dairy sector is of considerable economic importance. In March 1989 there were about 42,000 registered milk producers in the UK, compared with 200,000 in 1945. The total dairy cow population is 2.8 million and the average dairy herd size 65 — more than three times the size of the average unit within the EC. Milk together with milk products manufactured on farm accounted for 21% of total UK farm output in 1989, its value to farmers being £2.7 billion. In 1987, around 50,000 people were employed in milk product manufacture, representing about 10% of the total workforce in food manufacturing.

5.3 Also there are important import and export trades in milk products; imports were worth £747 million in 1988 (9% of UK food imports by value), and exports £370 million (10% of UK food exports). Cheese and butter are the most important products in both trades. Very little liquid milk is imported.

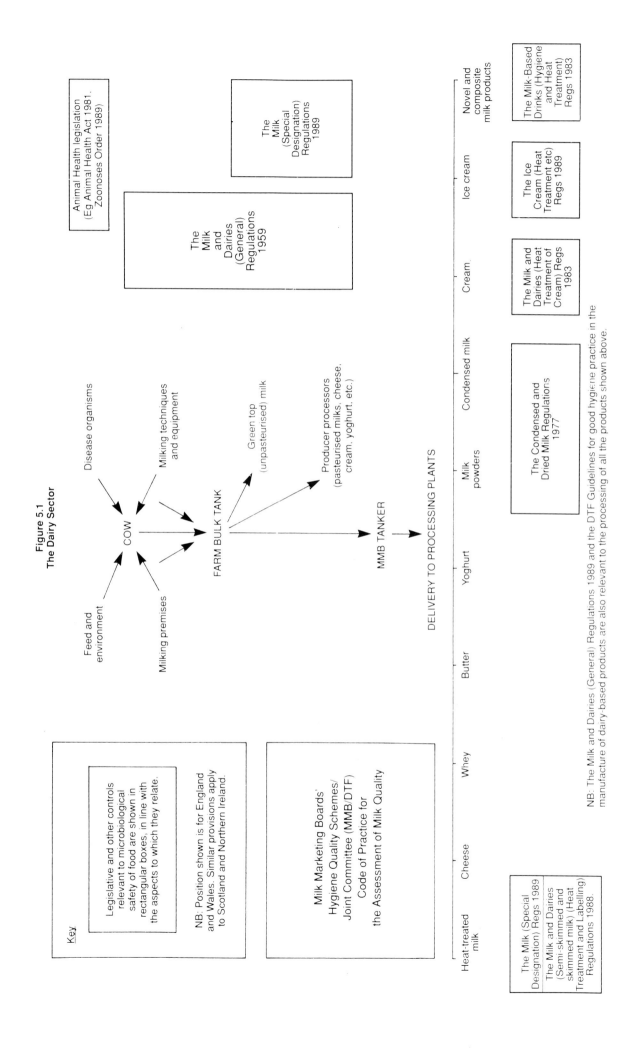

Figure 5.1
The Dairy Sector

Animal Health legislation
(Eg Animal Health Act 1981.
Zoonoses Order 1989)

The Milk (Special Designation) Regulations 1989

The Milk and Dairies (General) Regulations 1959

Disease organisms

Milking techniques and equipment

Feed and environment

Milking premises

COW

FARM BULK TANK

Green top (unpasteurised) milk

Producer processors (pasteurised milks, cheese, cream, yoghurt, etc.)

MMB TANKER

DELIVERY TO PROCESSING PLANTS

Key

Legislative and other controls relevant to microbiological safety of food are shown in rectangular boxes, in line with the aspects to which they relate.

NB: Position shown is for England and Wales. Similar provisions apply to Scotland and Northern Ireland.

Milk Marketing Boards' Hygiene Quality Schemes/ Joint Committee (MMB/DTF) Code of Practice for the Assessment of Milk Quality

Heat-treated milk
Cheese
Whey
Butter
Yoghurt
Milk powders
Condensed milk
Cream
Ice cream
Novel and composite milk products

The Milk (Special Designation) Regs 1989
The Milk and Dairies (Semi-skimmed and skimmed milk) (Heat Treatment and Labelling) Regulations 1988.

The Condensed and Dried Milk Regulations 1977

The Milk and Dairies (Heat Treatment of Cream) Regs 1983

The Ice Cream (Heat Treatment etc) Regs 1989

The Milk-Based Drinks (Hygiene and Heat Treatment) Regs 1983

NB: The Milk and Dairies (General) Regulations 1989 and the DTF Guidelines for good hygiene practice in the manufacture of dairy-based products are also relevant to the processing of all the products shown above.

5.4 Just over 14 billion litres of milk were produced in 1988/89. Table 5.1 below shows milk utilisation, according to the main product categories, in 1968/69 and 1988/89. Total production has increased, but consumption of liquid milk, cream and condensed milk has fallen. As a result, much larger volumes now go for butter and cheese production.

Table 5.1: **UK Milk Utilisation 1968/69 and 1988/89**

	1968/69		1988/89	
	Million litres	% of total	Million litres	% of total
Liquid market	7,474	64	6,760	48
Butter	1,237	10.5	2,822	20
Cheese	1,241	10.5	2,884	21
Condensed Milk (incl chocolate crumb)	627	5	420	3
Whole milk powder	214	2	541	4
Cream	759	7	485	3
Other	105	1	96	1
Total	11,657	100%	14,008	100%

Source: UK Dairy Facts and Figures 1969 and 1989

5.5 Consumer expenditure on milk and milk products was estimated to be £4.93 billion in 1989, or 12.6% of all household expenditure on food: a breakdown is shown in the table at Annex 5.1.

5.6 Milk is also an important element in the national diet. The National Food Survey shows for example that the average consumption of liquid milk in the home is approximately half a pint per person per day — some 24% above the average consumption elsewhere in the EC. Dairy products in total contribute significantly to the average daily intake of certain nutrients and total energy, providing 14% of energy, 22% of protein, 38% of riboflavin and 57% of calcium.

5.7 One particular feature of the sector is a small market for untreated liquid milk (i.e. raw milk which has not been pasteurised) sold to the public for direct consumption. Sale of milk in this way has been banned in Scotland since 1983. Untreated milk accounts for less than 1% of the liquid milk market. Goats' and sheep's milk are small but growing sectors of milk production. Background information on these sectors is set out at Annex 5.2.

INCIDENCE OF FOODBORNE DISEASE ASSOCIATED WITH MILK AND MILK PRODUCTS

5.8 Annex 5.3 sets out the information on outbreaks of foodborne disease which have been associated with milk and milk products during the period 1980-89. Of those linked with liquid milk, the majority have resulted from the consumption of untreated (raw) milk, and commonly involve infection with salmonella (particularly with *S.typhimurium.* a serotype especially associated with bovines) or campylobacter. In this connection it is interesting to note the reduction that occurred in milk-related foodborne infection in Scotland once the sale of untreated milk for direct consumption was banned in 1983. We examine issues relating to the consumption of untreated milk in paragraphs 5.25-5.29 below. The minority of outbreaks which have involved pasteurised milk were due to defective pasteurisation or to post-pasteurisation contamination and arose because of poor management in dairy plants; they emphasise the need for rigorous application of the Hazard Analysis Critical Control Point (HACCP) approach in pasteurisation plants. We comment further on the data in Annex 5.3 in the later sections of this chapter which deal with different milk products.

LEGISLATIVE PROVISIONS 5.9 The bovine dairy industry was among the first sectors of the food industry to be controlled by hygiene legislation. The original aim to control tuberculosis has long since been attained. However, legislation has developed over the years to encompass all aspects of hygienic production, with the European Community increasingly playing a leading role. Detailed domestic regulations (some of them implementing EC requirements) now cover all stages of cows' milk production and distribution, and the manufacture of many cows' milk products. There are also codes of practice from various different sources, which deal with hygiene control during the handling, production and sale of milk and milk products.

5.10 The main statutory requirements on milk and milk products which have a bearing on health and hygiene are summarised below and also in Figure 5.1. The provisions quoted cover England and Wales; separate provisions cover Scotland and Northern Ireland, but have broadly similar effect.

a. Production

5.11 The Milk and Dairies (General) Regulations 1959 (SI 1959 No 277) provide that:—

— all dairy farmers and all premises used for dairying (including milking parlours) must be registered;

— registration of premises is conditional upon the attainment of structural standards, the provision of safe and adequate water supplies, and the maintenance of effective hygienic equipment and milking routines;

— dairy farms are inspected periodically by MAFF, and may be de-registered if any breaches of the regulations are not swiftly corrected.

5.12 There is a prohibition, under Section 35 of the Food Act 1984, on the sale, or use for manufacture, of milk from cows suffering from "acute mastitis, actinomycosis of the udder, suppuration of the udder, any infection of the udder or teats which is likely to convey disease, any comatose condition, any septic condition of the uterus, anthrax, and foot-and-mouth disease".

b. Processing, storage and transport

5.13 The Milk (Special Designation) Regulations 1989 (SI 1989 No 2383) provide as follows:—

— processing dairies must be licensed to carry out pasteurisation, sterilisation or ultra heat treatment of milk. Enforcement of the regulations for heat treatment of milk in dairies is by qualified environmental health officers employed by the local authority;

— heat treatment plants must be equipped with temperature recording apparatus and, in the case of continuous flow systems, with flow diversion valves;

— microbiological standards are set for raw milk prior to treatment;

— the treatment processes are prescribed;

— microbiological standards are set for the heat-treated milk;

— special conditions are set under which untreated milk may be sold under licence for direct human consumption in England and Wales. (However, the sale of untreated milk in Scotland is banned — see paragraph 5.26 below).

5.14 The Milk and Dairies (General) Regulations 1959 also provide for:—

— dairies other than those on dairy farms to be registered. EHOs enforce these regulations in relation to the compliance by processing dairies with the structural and other hygiene standards specified;

— milk which is shown to be infected by disease communicable to man to be heat treated before being sold for human consumption.

c. Effect of Food Safety Act 1990

5.15 The Food Safety Act 1990 omits much of the detailed provision on milk and dairies contained in the Food Act 1984. We understand, however, that this, including the prohibition quoted in paragraph 5.12 above, will be transferred to the secondary legislation. Similarly the substance of existing regulations will be retained, including the heat treatment condition mentioned in paragraph 5.14 above. The regulations will, however, be reviewed in the light of the proposed Community legislation on milk hygiene (paragraphs 5.17 and 5.18 below).

5.16 Regulations are to be made under the Food Safety Act 1990 covering training requirements for those who handle food, which may include workers in milk processing establishments.

d. EC Legislation

5.17 A European Community Directive (85/397/EEC) applies to heat-treated milk traded between EC member states. Its provisions are comprehensive, and apply to all stages of the food chain for milk, from the farm to the consumer. It lays down two sets of microbiological standards for heat-treated milk. Member states who have satisfied the EC Commission that heat-treated milk for consumption on their domestic market is capable of meeting the higher Step 2 standard are entitled to apply that same standard to imports of heat-treated milk. Only the United Kingdom and Denmark have been recognised as achieving Step 2 status. The Step 2 microbiological standards for pasteurised milk are as follows:—

— that a sample of pasteurised milk gives a coliform count of less than one per ml;

— that a sample of pasteurised milk gives a plate count of not more than 30,000 per ml;

— that a sample of the pasteurised milk, after incubation for five days at 6°C, gives a plate count of not more than 100,000 per ml after the plated sample has been incubated for 25 hours at 21°C.

5.18 The EC Commission has issued a proposal (COM(89)672) which would convert the heat-treated milk directive into a regulation which would apply requirements to all heat-treated milk produced in the EC, rather than simply to intra-Community trade. However, as explained in paragraph 5.17 above, the stricter Step 2 microbiological standards set by the Directive already have to be met by heat-treated milk produced in, or imported into, the UK. There is a parallel EC Commission proposal (COM(89)667) for a regulation setting health rules (including microbiological standards) for the production, processing and manufacture of milk other than heat-treated cows' milk, and of milk products: it covers milk from cows, sheep, goats and buffaloes, and deals with raw milk, milk for manufacture, and milk-based products. These proposals form part of the programme for completing the internal market within the EC by 1993. As at November 1990, negotiations on them had yet to start in the EC Council of Ministers; however, the Government had consulted interested parties in preparation for negotiations.

e. Sheep's and goats' milk

5.19 The production of sheep's and goats' milk — or indeed the milk of other mammal species — has not hitherto been covered by detailed statutory controls in the same way as cows' milk, although voluntary codes of practice covering the hygienic production of these milks have been issued by the Government. The Food Safety Act 1990 has in our view remedied an important shortcoming by giving Ministers the power to make regulations on sheep's and goats' milk for the first time.

THE HYGIENIC QUALITY OF MILK MARKETED IN THE UK

5.20 The wholesale marketing of raw milk in the UK is arranged through five statutory Milk Marketing Boards (MMBs) (one for England and Wales, and the Scottish, the Aberdeen and District, the North of Scotland and the Northern Ireland MMBs). Over 98% of UK milk production which is available for human consumption goes through the MMBs' schemes. They have achieved considerable improvements in the quality of milk, in part by using their contracts with producers to impose a number of measures concerning milk production and handling, including the installation of bulk tanks on all farms and the requirement to cool milk to less than 4.5°C. Also, each of the MMBs has introduced payment schemes which apply financial incentives and penalties in relation to hygienic quality, milk composition, and antibiotic residues. An illustration of this is given in Annex 5.4 which shows the improvement in the total bacterial count (TBC) that resulted following the introduction in October 1982 of central testing and graduated financial penalties by the MMB (England and Wales). The MMB's incentives and penalties in relation to TBC can mean a difference of more than 50% in the price farmers receive for milk in the top and bottom categories.

5.21 The legislation described earlier, together with the rigorous application of controls and penalties by the MMBs, has enabled the hygienic quality of milk marketed in the UK to meet the highest standard specified in European Community legislation (see paragraph 5.17 above).

EXAMINATION OF THE LIQUID MILK PRODUCTION CHAIN (see Figure 5.1) Milk Production on the Farm

5.22 Dairy cows are typically kept at grass in summer and under cover in the winter, bedded on straw or shavings, most often with individual cubicles to lie in. Winter feeding is based on conserved grass in the form of silage or hay, supplemented with compound feed. Only good quality silage (ie with a pH below 5, well preserved and free from mould) should be fed to milking cows. Silage is a potential source of listeriosis in cattle, which can result in the excretion of *Listeria spp* in the milk (see our comments at Part I, Appendix 3, paragraph A.3.5). As clinical cases are readily diagnosed (cf Part II, paragraph 4.21), such milk does not enter the food chain.

5.23 Milk is well suited to the growth of microorganisms. It is therefore essential that handling and milking techniques minimise the risks of contamination by bacteria from the environment and from the cow's urine, faeces, bedding and feedingstuffs. Husbandry and cow health are of paramount importance in relation to the microbiological standard of milk. The Committee has identified the following stages in the process as important areas (see also Annex 5.5):—

a. microbiological quality of feed;

b. suitability of housing (in particular, design of lying areas to reduce soiling of udder and teats and to keep bedding clean and dry);

c. regular replacement of bedding, and cleaning of feeding areas;

d. maintenance of udder health and cleanliness (through washing and drying of udder before milking, checking for infection, discarding fore milk);

e. hand washing and other hygienic measures by milking personnel;

f. discarding of milk from cows showing symptoms of, or under treatment for, udder disease;

g. sanitisation of milking parlour equipment, after each milking, with approved chemical solutions;

h. regular maintenance of equipment to obviate teat-end damage;

i. effective sanitisation of the bulk tank and temperature control of its contents;

j. regular testing of the water supply.

5.24 These potential hazard areas in the production of milk have long been recognised. The range of control measures we have outlined, together with the MMBs' hygienic quality schemes, has enabled UK milk production generally to achieve very high standards of hygiene. Every effort must be made to ensure that these standards are maintained.

Liquid Raw Milk

5.25 As noted in paragraph 5.7 above, a small amount of cows' milk is sold untreated for direct consumption. There is also a small trade in goats' and sheep's milk, much of it in frozen form.

5.26 Annex 5.3 highlights the impact of pasteurisation of milk on the incidence of foodborne disease in two very clear ways:—

— by far the majority of outbreaks are associated with untreated milk;

— following the introduction from 1983 of the ban of the sale in Scotland of liquid untreated milk for direct consumption, a sharp drop occurred in the number of cases of food poisoning in Scotland associated with milk consumption. (The ban was extended in 1986 to cover the giving of untreated milk to agricultural workers as a wage-benefit).

5.27 Part I, Annex 9.3 records that on 12 June 1989 we wrote to Ministers drawing attention to the hazards involved in the consumption of untreated milk. Our comments were made in the context that the then Minister of Agriculture, Fisheries and Food was conducting a consultation on a proposal to ban the sale of untreated milk in England and Wales for direct consumption, in the same way as had already been applied in Scotland. As a result of the consultation, Ministers decided that consumers in England and Wales should continue to be allowed to decide for themselves whether or not to drink untreated milk, but should be made aware of the risks involved through the introduction of more explicit labelling requirements. In addition, in order to help ensure health risks are minimised, more rigorous microbiological standards were introduced.

5.28 Having considered milk and milk product manufacture in detail, the Committee now repeats its strongly-held view that consumption of untreated milk is hazardous. The hazard primarily concerns salmonella and campylobacter infections: however, we note (see Annex 5.3) that a particularly serious outbreak occurred in Yorkshire in 1984 as a result of the contamination of raw milk with *Streptococcus zooepidemicus;* twelve people were admitted to hospital, of whom eight died. The effect of the outbreak was probably heightened by the fact that nine of those affected were over 70 and one was an infant of one day old. This episode well illustrates why we are concerned at the continuing consumption of raw milk. **We recommend that the Government's new measures relating to the testing and labelling of untreated milk should be very rigorously enforced and the incidence of foodborne illness associated with the consumption of untreated milk kept closely under review** (R(II)5.1).

5.29 As we have noted, the production of sheep's and goats' milk is a small but growing activity, which involves some sale of untreated liquid milk direct to the consumer, and which has hitherto not been subject to detailed regulatory control. We welcome the fact that the Government has taken powers to make such regulations through the Food Safety Act 1990, and the fact that the EC proposal (COM(89)667) for a Regulation on milk products covers caprine and ovine products. **We recommend to the Government that milk and milk products originating from sheep and goats should be subjected as soon as possible to controls similar to those which apply to cows' milk and products made from it** (R(II)5.2).

Heat-Treated Liquid Milk (ie full fat, semi-skimmed and skimmed milks)

5.30 The heat treatment processes legally required for pasteurised, UHT and sterilised milk are described in Annex 5.6. Pasteurisation destroys a very high proportion of the vegetative pathogenic organisms present in raw milk (for example, about 6 decimal reductions for salmonella), but clearly some organisms will survive if they are originally present in high enough numbers. It is therefore essential that raw milk should be of the highest quality possible.

5.31 In the UHT process the milk, after heat treatment (direct or indirect) to a temperature in excess of 135°C for one second, is processed and packaged under aseptic conditions. In the sterilisation process, milk is usually given an initial heat treatment, packaged and then given a further heat treatment in the container. No cases of infection have been associated with UHT or sterilised milk (see Annex 5.3).

5.32 The reception of raw milk by the processing plant is an important control point since the risk exists of introducing pathogenic organisms into the site via either the vehicle or the milk. Appropriate design of the site itself will reduce the former hazard while tests carried out on the milk will reduce the latter. The standards and tests for raw milk arriving at a dairy by tanker are set out in the Code of Practice for the Assessment of Milk Quality agreed by the Joint Committee of the Milk Marketing Board and the Dairy Trade Federation. A number of tests are carried out on each tanker load on arrival, with a view to obtaining results before the consignment is accepted for processing. These usually include temperature, freezing point depression, organoleptic qualities, composition (fat and other solids) and the 10 minute Resazurin Test that detects heavy contamination with bacteria. Very few tanker loads (well under 1%) have to be rejected on the basis of these tests. High milk temperature (>7°C) and low freezing point depression are the main reasons for failure.

5.33 In addition to the rapid tests, other tests for antibiotics, acidity, total viable count and thermoduric count are also undertaken by the receiving dairy at less frequent intervals (weekly or more often, depending on local factors). Any results exceeding the standards laid down in the Joint Committee Code are reported to the local MMB marketing officer, who will undertake the necessary investigations to improve the raw milk quality. We are satisfied that this system of checks provides an effective means of screening tanker loads of milk on arrival at the processing plant.

5.34 The critical points in the pasteurisation process have been highlighted in Annex 5.7. Pasteurisation is an effective process if it is carried out properly. Failures of the process are extremely rare, but it is nonetheless vital to take careful precautions to prevent them; breakdown in the pasteurisation process could potentially cause problems for a very large number of people. A problem area of particular importance is cleaning and maintenance of pasteurisation plant, including pipelines. Plant often appears not to have been designed with cleanability in mind, and equipment manufacturers do not commonly issue instructions on cleaning arrangements and procedures. Users are left to devise the cleaning arrangements themselves, and often experience difficulty in getting manufacturers to take notice of their requirements.

5.35 Where contamination of milk occurs after pasteurisation, the most common causes are inadequately washed bottles and poor cleaning of the fillers. This stems primarily from the same problems with the cleaning and maintenance of machinery as have been noted in paragraph 5.34.

5.36 **We recommend that designers of equipment for heat treatment and bottling — including pipelines — should take proper account of the needs of hygiene, and especially of the need to enable in-place cleaning to be undertaken if at all possible** (R(II)5.3).

EXAMINATION OF THE PRODUCTION CHAIN FOR CHEESE
The Sector

5.37 Just over 20% of UK milk supplies are used for cheese manufacture. The UK retail cheese market was estimated to be worth about £1,140m in 1989 (Source: National Food Survey). There is a trend towards more expensive (and often imported) cheeses. Estimated retail sales in 1989 were 329,000 tonnes of which hard cheeses (eg cheddar) accounted for 81%. Soft mould-ripened cheeses at present account for about 10% of the market and are taking an increasing share.

5.38 We consider the main controls for cheese production to be (see also the flow charts at Annexes 5.8 and 5.9):—

— use milk of high microbiological standard;

— use starter cultures from a reliable source;

— monitor acid development during fermentation, isolate any products from slow fermentations, and test for pathogens and indicator organisms;

— monitor environment and product for total counts and pathogens;

— apply high standards of hygiene at all times.

5.39 **We recommend to producers the detailed advice on production of soft cheese which is set out in "Guidelines for good hygienic practice in the manufacture of soft and fresh cheeses", which was produced by the Creamery Proprietors' Association in 1988** (R(II)5.4). These have been incorporated into the Dairy Trade Federation's "Guidelines for good hygienic practice in the manufacture of dairy based products". The guidelines specify and recommend hygienic principles for cheese manufacture and the HACCP approach.

5.40 Reported incidents of foodborne illness attributed to milk products in the UK include a few associated with cheese. Annex 5.3 shows that between 1980 and 1989 there have been four outbreaks of staphylococcal food poisoning and one of salmonellosis; there have also been two sporadic cases of listeriosis associated with soft cheese consumption, one involving cheese imported from France, and the other a UK-produced goats' milk cheese. In the past decade, therefore, despite the very substantial size of the cheese sector, very few recorded outbreaks of foodborne illness have been attributed to cheese.

5.41 Typical manufacturing processes for hard cheese and for soft mould-ripened cheeses are outlined in Annexes 5.8 and 5.9. Many variations on these typical processes exist, and it is therefore extremely difficult to generalise. However, the cheese-making process normally begins with a lactic acid fermentation which results in an accumulation of lactic acid and a decrease in pH. The main differences between hard and mould-ripened cheeses which affect microbiological stability are as follows:—

Hard cheeses (includes cheeses whose curds have been subjected to significant pressure during production, eg cheddar, cheshire and lancashire)

>   low water activity
>   low pH
>   high salt content

Mould-ripened cheese (includes cheeses ripened by the action of moulds and/or bacteria, eg brie, stilton and camembert)

>   high water activity
>   high pH
>   low salt content

Cottage cheese and similar products are normally short shelf-life products, have a low pH (<pH 5.0), and as such will present a low microbiological risk if properly made from high quality raw materials.

5.42 During the maturation of hard cheeses the combination of high salt, high acidity and low water activity of the cheese with a long maturation time are unfavourable to the survival of most pathogens. Thus, proper attention to hygiene during the manufacturing process leads to a microbiologically safe product.

5.43 In mould-ripened cheese, ripening occurs through the growth of moulds and bacteria on the surface and inside the cheese. The growth of these organisms raises the pH of the cheese to levels significantly in excess of pH 5.0; under such conditions contaminating organisms can grow. With such cheeses, the risk of contamination is increased through exposure of the cheese to the environment during the maturation process.

5.44 PHLS surveys in 1986 and 1989 of soft mould-ripened cheeses obtained mainly from retail outlets found that 8-10% of the cheeses were contaminated with *L.monocytogenes*. The levels were normally low but in a few samples counts exceeding 10^5 cfu/g were found. The contamination rates for cheeses made with pasteurised and untreated milks were similar, suggesting that the source of the contamination was principally environmental.

5.45 As described in Part I, paragraphs 2.12 and 2.13, listeria organisms are widely distributed in the environment, so that exposure to these bacteria is unavoidable.

L.monocytogenes is reported to be present in the gastointestinal tract of around 1 in 20 of the healthy human population at any one time. Surveillance has indicated that the disease listeriosis is rare. There were 291 cases in 1988, and 250 in 1989. As noted above (Part II, paragraph 1.18), a significant reduction has occurred in the first six months of 1990, with 58 cases being recorded compared with 156 in the equivalent period in 1989. It is possible that cases of listeriosis involving no more than a mild flu-like illness are frequently undiagnosed, but the cases reported to the PHLS often involve septicaemia or meningitis and the fatality rate is around 30%. Although the disease in the pregnant woman is usually mild, the consequences can include abortion, stillbirth, or listeriosis in the newborn baby.

5.46 In February 1989 the Government's Chief Medical Officer (CMO) issued advice in the following terms:—

> "...having taken the best possible expert advice, I would advise that pregnant women should avoid eating certain types of soft cheeses. It is not possible to specify precisely the cheeses in which Listeria is likely to grow, but on the basis of current information these are likely to be soft ripened cheeses such as the brie, camembert, and blue vein types. On the other hand, hard cheeses such as the cheddar and cheshire types, processed cheeses, cottage cheeses and cheese spreads have not given cause for concern."

The CMO also advised that, as well as pregnant women, "those with underlying illness which results in impaired resistance to infection, such as patients who have had transplants, those on particular drugs which depress the immune system and those with leukemia or cancers of the lymphatic tissues" should also follow this advice. The CMO's advice is reproduced in full at Annex 5.10.

5.47 Under a "gentlemen's agreement" reached among the EC member states in December 1987, an agreed detection method must be used for sampling cheeses for *L.monocytogenes*. The terms of the agreement state that the finding of positive results at the point of manufacture shall lead to more intensive sampling and sanitising. When cheese already marketed is found to be positive for *L.monocytogenes*, the agreement provides for tracing-back to the premises of origin and the taking of sanitising measures there; where applicable, for the direct transmission of information to the authorities in the member state of origin and to the EC Commission; and for the withdrawal from the market of the batch concerned if it is considered to be a danger to human health. The EC Commission has proposed in effect that this informal agreement should be overtaken by binding legal requirements, since the microbiological standards proposed for inclusion in the intended EC regulation on milk products (see paragraph 5.18 above) would include one applicable to cheese.

5.48 We consider that the effective operation of this gentlemen's agreement, or of any successor to it, logically depends on the setting of standards which can be agreed as the basis for withdrawal action. Consequently we welcome the fact that the European Community is to address this question by virtue of its inclusion in the Commission's proposal, and **we recommend the Government to work for the adoption of a well-founded and practical standard for the presence of *L.monocytogenes* in cheese which can be worked to and enforced internationally** (R(II)5.5).

Cheeses made from untreated milk

5.49 There has been some public debate about the safety of this type of cheese. We note that the number of outbreaks of foodborne illness that have been associated with cheese made from untreated milk is very small; Annex 5.3 shows the following since 1980:—

1984 — outbreak (in Scotland) associated with Staphylococcal enterotoxin in sheep's milk cheese;

1985 — outbreak (in Scotland) associated with Staphylococcal enterotoxin in sheep's milk cheese;

1988 — outbreak of unknown cause, but presumed to be due to Staphylococcal enterotoxin, in cheese made from unpasteurised milk;

1989 — outbreak associated with Salmonella dublin in cheese imported from Ireland.

5.50 The main microbiological hazards associated with making cheese from untreated milk are:—

a. a failure of hygiene at early control points in the chain (animal husbandry and milking, handling and transportation), which may result in the milk used as raw material being contaminated with faecal organisms such as salmonella;

b. the possible carryover of microorganisms in milk arising from cows affected by sub-acute mastitis, eg *Staph.aureus* and occasionally *L.monocytogenes;*

c. the possible introduction of pathogens into the milk from the environment.

The use of untreated milk for cheese manufacture means that the raw material has not been subjected to a heat treatment capable of eliminating harmful microorganisms that may have entered in any of the ways shown above. The microbiological safety of cheese made from untreated milk therefore depends on the efficiency of the remaining control steps, ie the development of acid during fermentation and the prevention of contamination during processing. The efficiency of these is monitored by (a) measuring the acidity during fermentation and (b) monitoring for total bacterial and specific pathogen counts in the end product.

5.51 **We recommend that Government should ensure at both the national and European levels that cheese producers are made fully aware of the microbiological hazards of making cheese from untreated milk; that strict hygienic controls are laid down for the production of cheese, including monitoring the microbiological standard of the milk used; and that every step be taken through the application of the HACCP approach and end product monitoring to ensure that the cheese is microbiologically safe and is not contaminated after processing (R(II)5.6).**

5.52 We note the statement of 24 August 1990 from the Food Minister that he is exploring with other EC member states the possibililty of building into the harmonised food labelling rules a requirement concerning the labelling of cheese made from unpasteurised milk. Such a requirement would be of assistance to consumers who wish to know, when purchasing cheese, whether it is made from pasteurised or unpasteurised milk.

EXAMINATION OF THE PRODUCTION CHAIN FOR OTHER MILK PRODUCTS

5.53 Chapter 7 of the first part of our report contains a thorough appraisal of manufacturing processes in general, including an account of the HACCP approach. A very wide range of food products is derived from milk, including cheese, dried products (skimmed and full fat powders), yoghurt, cream, butter, ice cream and novel milk and composite milk products (see Figure 5.1 above). Many of the more traditional products are covered by compositional regulations, supplemented in some cases by heat treatment requirements (eg cream, ice cream). Milk products have not been a major cause of food poisoning in recent years. There have been a few well publicised outbreaks which have occurred because of poor hygiene practices. In the paragraphs below we focus briefly on those products where we feel there are points to be made.

Milk Powders
(see flowchart at Annex 5.11)

5.54 Milk powders have occasionally caused outbreaks including some in the UK. The most recent reported UK outbreak (see Annex 5.3) was caused in 1985 by contamination of infant formula with *Salmonella ealing* and involved 62 cases, including one death. The outbreak was attributed to contaminated powder deposits in the insulation of the spray drier reaching the product through cracks in the drier. This is an illustration of how a small defect can have wide-ranging effects. After this outbreak the UK dairy trade, through the Creamery Proprietors' Association, used the HACCP approach to produce guidelines on hygienic production of milk powders. Following this code of practice should prevent future problems. Poor design and maintenance of drying equipment is known to have been a contributory factor in contamination of milk powders. **We recommend that ways of improving the design of driers and ancillary equipment used in the manufacture of milk powder be investigated** (R(II)5.7).

Yoghurt
(see flowchart at Annex 5.12)

5.55 Yoghurt does not in itself present a food poisoning hazard as its low pH prevents the growth of pathogens and toxin production. The incident in 1989 in which 27 cases of botulism, including one death, arose from consumption of hazelnut yoghurt was caused by the addition to the yoghurt base of an inadequately heat processed hazelnut puree, rather than by any problem involving the yoghurt itself. The incident shows not only that the manufacturers of food and food ingredients must have a proper appreciation of the microbiological hazards of their activities, but also that those who use food ingredients should take steps to assure themselves of the microbiological safety of those ingredients.

Ice cream
(see flowchart at Annex 5.13)

5.56 Regulations were introduced in 1947 which, for the first time, required the heat treatment of all ice cream mixes. The current version of the Regulations is the Ice Cream (Heat Treatment etc) Regulations 1959. The result of this heat treatment prior to the freezing of the mix is that ice cream is no longer a significant cause of foodborne disease. Recent suggestions that high levels of bacterial contamination can occur are related to alleged poor hygiene by some vendors: this point is dealt with in our chapter on retailing (Part II, Chapter 8).

Butter
(see flowchart at Annex 5.14)

5.57 Milk used to produce butter is normally pasteurised before separation. In addition, most butter in the UK does not present a food safety problem because it has a low water activity due to a high salt content in the water phase. However, reduced fat butter is less stable — see paragraph 5.59 below.

Novel and composite milk products

5.58 The dairy industry manufactures a range of novel foods based on traditional milk-based products. These include reduced or low fat butter, low fat and fresh cheeses, yoghurts containing a range of fruit and vegetable pieces, and processed cheeses containing meat, fish and vegetable pieces. There is also a wide range of powdered milk-based drinks and flavoured heat-sterilised milk products.

5.59 Low fat butters are potentially more microbiologically unstable than natural butter because of their increased water content and the generally coarser dispersion of the water phase droplets in the fat phase. Stability is achieved by, for instance, the use of salt and organic acids in the water phase to control the growth of contaminating microorganisms. This is often combined with pasteurisation and followed by an emulsification with the fat phase under very carefully controlled conditions so that the final product will be free of pathogenic microorganisms or spore-formers which have not been killed. These products have to be refrigerated during distribution, sale and storage before use.

5.60 The addition of pieces of fruit, nuts or vegetable materials to high water activity cheeses and yoghurts that are normally stable as a result of their acidity may reduce the shelf-life of these products. Their use should therefore be carefully controlled by the manufacturer. Any ingredients added must be of the highest microbiological quality and treated in such a way as not to add organisms capable of growth in the food products. Hence canned or otherwise processed products are used. The filling/mixing must also be done under very clean conditions.

5.61 The addition of pieces of meat, of vegetable or of other ingredients can also reduce the safety of low water activity foods. For example processed cheese with added onion was responsible for an outbreak of botulism in Argentina. Processed cheeses are heat treated and are stable at ambient temperatures provided that they have a high solids content, low water activity and high acidity. The composition of the processed cheese prevents the growth of any spore-forming bacteria (eg *Clostridium botulinum*) that may survive the heat treatment. Vegetable pieces and similar ingredients often have a lower solids content, a higher water activity and a higher pH, and will support the growth of spore formers. To ensure the stability of composite products, control measures must be taken, eg marinading or sterilising the added ingredients.

5.62 Many novel milk-based products are attractive to the consumer, and sound techniques exist for their safe production. However, safe processes are in many cases microbiologically demanding, and **we recommend that manufacturers should ensure that the production of novel and composite milk products is always subject to expert assessment and close monitoring** (R(II)5.8).

ANNEX 5.1

MILK AND MILK PRODUCTS: NATIONAL CONSUMPTION AND EXPENDITURE 1989

	Estimated		Estimated UK Consumer Expenditure on food consumed in home	
	(a) Household Consumption (per person per week)	(b) Household Expenditure (pence per person per week)	(£ million)	Total (£bn)
MILK				
UHT liquid wholemilk	0.02 pints	0.52	15	
Sterilised wholemilk	0.12 "	3.60	103	
Other wholemilk				
(incl pasteurised, homogenised)	2.23 "	60.45	1,723	
Welfare milk	0.04 "	—	—	
School milk	0.01 "	0.10	3	
Fully skimmed milk	0.34 "	8.91	254	
Semi and other skimmed milk	0.76 "	20.61	587	2.69
CHEESE				
Hard: cheddar & cheddar type	2.50 oz	23.49	669	
other UK varieties or				
foreign equivalents	0.53 "	5.28	150	
edam & other continental	0.27 "	2.88	82	
Soft	0.46 "	4.82	137	
Processed cheese	0.31 "	3.54	101	1.14
BUTTER				
New Zealand butter	0.43 oz	2.84	81	
Danish butter	0.34 "	2.41	69	
UK butter	0.45 "	3.03	86	
All other butter	0.54 "	3.51	100	0.34
OTHER				
Other milk				
(buttermilk, goats', sourmilk, souffle,				
syllabub, fresh cream desserts)	0.04 pints	3.45	98	
Condensed milk	0.06 "(equivalent)	1.63	46	
Infant formula	0.05 "(equivalent)	1.81	52	
Instant milk	0.07 "(equivalent)	1.37	39	
Yoghurt	0.16 "	14.09	402	
Cream	0.03 "	4.30	123	0.76
			Grand Total	4.93

Source: National Food Survey
MAFF

ANNEX 5.2

PRODUCTION OF GOATS' AND SHEEP'S MILK

5.2.1. Goats' milk, although a small sector, is a developing one. The census of June 1989 suggested that there were some 23,400 goats on 4,563 agricultural holdings (other than minor holdings) in England and Wales. Approximately 80% of these had fewer than five goats. However, a small number of producers operated on a more significant scale: 40 producers had around 100 goats each, and four had more than 400. The population of goats outside the scope of the census — eg on minor agricultural holdings and in back gardens — is unknown but likely to be as many again. In Scotland 48 milking goat herds have been identified and eight in Northern Ireland.

5.2.2. For sheep's milk, the census does not separately identify milk sheep, but the British Sheep Dairying Association has indicated that there are some 11,000 milking sheep in England and Wales, in approximately 230 flocks, distributed as follows:

30-35 sheep — 200 flocks

100-200 sheep — 20 flocks

over 200 sheep — 10 flocks

In Scotland seven milk sheep flocks have been identified, one with fewer than 20 sheep, five between 20 and 50 and one with over 400. The single sheep milking flock in Northern Ireland has 300-350 sheep.

ANNEX 5.3

OUTBREAKS OF FOODBORNE DISEASE ASSOCIATED WITH MILK AND MILK PRODUCTS
Confirmed Reports to CDSC, England and Wales 1980-1989

Year	Organism	Vehicle of infection	No. of outbreaks	Number affected (deaths)
1980	Salmonellas			
	S.typhimurium	raw milk	11	47
	S.typhimurium	goats' cheese	1	6
	Campylobacter sp	raw milk	5	163
	Campylocacter sp	pasteurised milk	1	30
			18	246
1981	Salmonellas			
	S.typhimurium	raw milk	10	59
	S.virchow	raw milk	3	12
	S.newport	raw milk	1	10
	Campylobacter sp	raw milk	7	213
	Staph. aureus	cream	1	25
	C. perfringens	milk poweder	1	77
			23	396
1982	Salmonellas			
	S.typhimurium	raw milk	14	409 (3)
	S.montevideo	raw milk	1	3
	Campylobacter sp	raw milk	3	200
	Campylobacter sp	pasteurised milk	1	400
			19	1,012
1983	Salmonellas			
	S.typhimurium	raw milk	5	198
	S.typhimurium	pasteurised milk	1	5
	S.typhimurium	cream**	1	2
	Campylobacter sp	raw milk	3	85
	Staph.aureus	cheese from pasteurised milk	1	2
			11	292
1984	Salmonellas			
	S.typhimurium	raw milk	11	301
	S.oranienburg	raw milk	1	12
	S.enteritidis	ice cream	1	12
	Campylobacter sp	raw milk	3	76
	Campylobacter	raw goats' milk	1	3
	Strep.zooepidemicus	raw milk	1	12 (8)
	Y.enterocolitica	pasteurised milk	1	2
			19	418
1985	Salmonellas			
	S.typhimurium	raw milk	5	49
	S.enteritidis	raw milk	1	5
	S.ealing	powdered milk	1	62
	Campylobacter sp	raw milk	6	178
	Y.enterocolitica	pasteurised milk	1	3
	unknown aetiology	pasteurised cream	1	16
	Staph.aureus	cheese (presumed from pasteurised milk)	1	28
			16	342

Year	Organism	Vehicle of infection	No. of outbreaks	Number affected (deaths)
*1986	Salmonellas			
	S.typhimurium	raw milk	3	316 (1)
	S.typhimurium	pasteurised cream	1	24
	S.braenderup	raw milk	1	5
	S.braenderup	pasteurised milk	1	39 (1)
	S.indiana	raw milk	1	2
	Campylobacter sp	raw milk	3	24
			10	410
*1987	Salmonellas			
	S.typhimurium	raw milk	2	31
	S.thielallee	raw milk	1	3
	Campylobacter sp	raw milk	6	332
	Campylobacter sp	pasteurised milk	2	526
	Campylobacter sp	milk shake	1	37
	B.cereus	ice cream	1	6
			13	935
*1988	Salmonellas			
	S.typhimurium	raw milk	2	7
	S.newport	raw milk	1	20
			3	27
†*1989	*S.dublin*	cheese (from unpasteurised milk)	1	39
	Campylobacter sp	milk**	1	14
	C.botulinum	hazelnut yoghurt	1	27 (1)
	Unknown	cheese (from unpasteurised milk)	1	155
			4	235

Source: PHLS Communicable Disease Surveillance Centre

*　　Unpublished data
**　Not known whether raw or pasteurised
†　　Provisional data

Note: two incidents concerning *L.monocytogenes*, in 1986 and 1988, were single cases, and so do not count as outbreaks.

OUTBREAKS OF FOODBORNE DISEASE ASSOCIATED WITH MILK AND MILK PRODUCTS
Confirmed Reports to Communicable Diseases (Scotland) Unit 1980-89

Year	Organism	Vehicle of infection	No. of outbreaks	Number affected (deaths)
1980	Salmonellas			
	S.typhimurium	raw milk	2	43 (3)
	S.virchow	raw milk	1	55 (1)
	Campylobacter sp	milk shake	1	4
			4	102
1981	Salmonellas			
	S.typhimurium	raw milk	5	679 (3)
	S.virchow	raw milk	1	32
	S.agona	raw milk	1	18
	Campylobacter sp	raw milk	1	53
			8	782
1982	S.typhimurium	raw milk	10	318 (1)
	Campylobacter sp	raw milk	4	221
			14	539
1983*	S.typhimurium	raw milk	4	21
	Campylobacter sp	raw milk	2	6
	Staph.enterotoxin	goats' milk (raw)	1	2
			7	29
1984	S.typhimurium	raw milk	4	25
	E.coli	raw cream	1	2
	Staph.enterotoxin	sheep's milk cheese	1	19
			6	46
1985	Salmonellas			
	S.typhimurium	raw milk	6	25
	S.dublin	raw milk	1	30
	Staph.enterotoxin	sheep's milk cheese	1	12
	Campylobacter sp	raw milk	1	19
			9	86
1986†	S.typhimurium	raw milk	1	4
	S.bovis-morbificans	raw milk	1	6
			2	10
1987	S.typhimurium	raw milk	2	7
	Campylobacter sp	raw milk	3	23
			5	30
1988	S.typhimurium	raw milk	1	4
			1	4
1989	—	—	—	—

* The Milk (Special Designation) (Scotland) Order 1980, was implemented on 1 August 1983.
† The Agricultural Wages Order No 34 (under the Agricultural Wages (Scotland) Act 1949), was implemented on 1 September 1986.

Note

There were two sporadic incidents in 1980-89 associated with raw milk. In 1980 a case of *Salmonella heidelberg* infection was confirmed by isolation of the organism from the child, milk and dairy cattle; but no further cases were identified among other consumers of the milk. In 1988 there was a case of Campylobacter enteritis in a child who consumed raw milk while on holiday on the Island of Colonsay, where only untreated milk was available at the villa. (This island had an exemption, renewable annually to sell raw cow's milk).

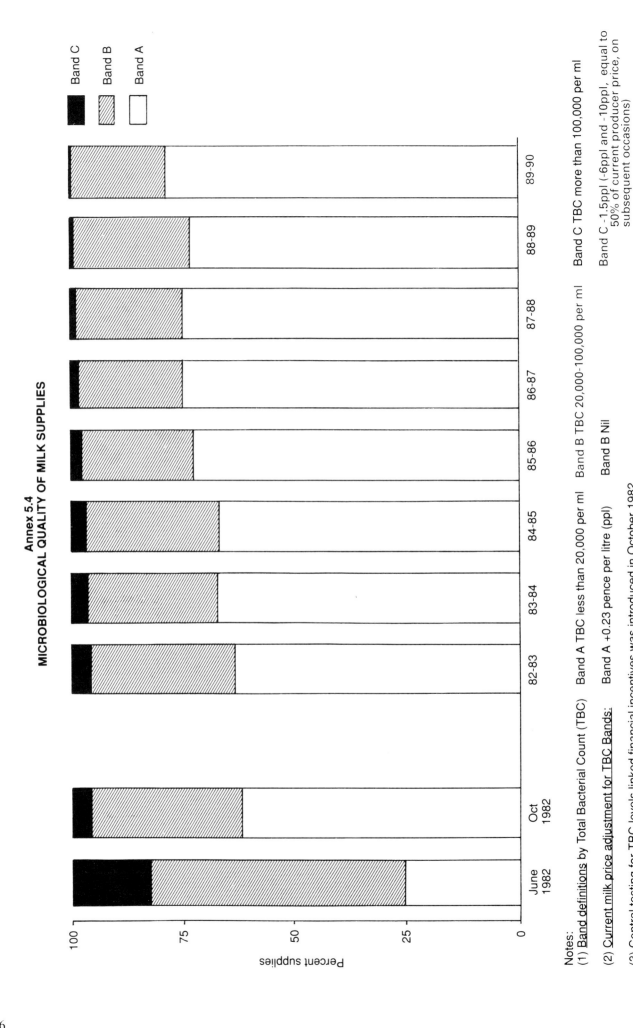

Annex 5.4
MICROBIOLOGICAL QUALITY OF MILK SUPPLIES

Notes:

(1) <u>Band definitions</u> by Total Bacterial Count (TBC)   Band A TBC less than 20,000 per ml   Band B TBC 20,000-100,000 per ml   Band C TBC more than 100,000 per ml

(2) <u>Current milk price adjustment for TBC Bands:</u>   Band A +0.23 pence per litre (ppl)   Band B Nil   Band C -1.5ppl (-6ppl and -10ppl, equal to 50% of current producer price, on subsequent occasions)

(3) Central testing for TBC levels linked financial incentives was introduced in October 1982.

ANNEX 5.5

MILK ON THE FARM: DAIRY HUSBANDRY CRITICAL POINTS FOR CONTAMINATION

Key event	Risk centre	Sanitisation Procedures
Dairy cow housing and holding areas	Contamination of udder and teats by environmental bacteria (mainly from bedding, urine, faeces).	Correctly designed lying area reduces soiling (of udder and teats) and keeps bedding clean and dry. Good management/husbandry ensures bedding is replaced when necessary and that feeding areas are cleaned regularly.
Cow in milking parlour	Contamination of udder and teats by environmental bacteria as above * udder washing and drying * discarded milk * milking personnel (esp. hands).	Floor, walls and external parts of milking equipment are cleaned after every milking. Udder washed and dried (using approved chemicals). Discarded milk is removed from contact with the bulk supply and from contact with other cows. Milking personnel wash hands (or rubber gloves if worn) before milking and after handling cows with infections, using approved cleansing agents. Water supply, if not mains, subject to regular testing.
Milk entering teat cup	Contaminated environment and bacteria from udder infections.	Teats cleaned before milking. Udder checked for infection before milking. Infected milk discarded.
Milking equipment	Multiplication of bacteria encouraged by inadequate cleaning, poor physical condition (especially rubber components) or bad design.	Cleaned after each milking with approved chemical solutions, and brushing where appropriate, followed by clean water rinse.
Bulk tank	Multiplication of bacteria encouraged by inadequate cleaning, inadequate cooling, poor physical condition.	After emptying, cleaned daily using approved chemical solution and brush, followed by clean water rinse.

ANNEX 5.6

HEAT TREATMENT OF MILK: RELEVANT REQUIREMENTS AND EFFECT ON MILK QUALITY

Requirements on plant design and operation

5.6.1. The design and operation of milk heat treatment plants are governed by legislation in most countries although details differ. In the UK all continuous flow heat treatment systems must have a flow diversion valve which automatically diverts the flow of inadequately processed milk and prevents contamination of the heat treated product. Operation of the valve is automatically recorded and these records have to be kept for at least three months. The other main requirements are summarised in Table 5.6.1 below. Full details are given in The Milk (Special Designation) Regulations 1989 (SI No 2383).*

5.6.2. Proper operation of the pasteurisation plant in accordance with the guidelines given, in the DTF Code of Practice and National Dairyman's Association Guidelines for the Safe Operation of Milk Pasteurisation, should ensure the safety of the final product.

Effects on Milk Quality

5.6.3. Heat treatment affects milk's chemical and physical properties in different ways according to the level of heat treatment. These effects are summarised in Table 5.6.2 below.

*Similar requirments exist in Scotland and Northern Ireland.

Table 5.6.1:
Legal requirements for heat processing

Product	Minimum time/temperature combinations	Other requirements
Pasteurised	b. 30 minutes at between 62.8°C and 65.6°C a. 15 seconds at 71.7°C	Milk must — be cooled immediately after heat treatment — be phosphatase negative — meet the microbiological standards — be packaged as soon as possible after pasteurisation. Records of heat treatment and cooling must be kept for at least 3 months.
UHT	1 sec at 135°C	Milk must — be packaged immediately into sterile containers under aseptic conditions. — meet the microbiological standards. Records of heat treatment must be kept for at least 3 months.
Sterilised	>100°C	Milk must — comply with turbidity test — meet microbiological standards. Records of heat treatment must be kept for at least 3 months.

Table 5.6.2:
Effect of heat treatment on milk

Process	Effect
Pasteurisation	Vitamin C — reduced by about 20% Thiamin ⎱ reduced by about 10% Vitamin B12 ⎰ slight disaggregation of fat globules resulting in reduced cream line — no nutritional significance.
UHT ⎱ Sterilised ⎰	Vitamin losses are greater than for pasteurised.

Note
1. Other minor changes occur to protein structure, enzyme, activities and calcium solubility.
2. These changes do not have a significant effect on dietary intakes of vitamin C, B12 and thiamin since milk is not an important source of these vitamins.

ANNEX 5.7

PRODUCTION OF PASTEURISED MILK

PROCESS	PROBLEM	ACTION
Arrival of raw milk	Raw milk may be contaminated with pathogens.	Check bacteriological quality of milk. Keep separate from areas where processed product handled.
Storage in silo, e.g. at ≤5°C	Some bacteria present will be able to grow.	Limit time in silo and ensure thorough cleaning after milk removed.
Pasteurisation (e.g. high temperature/short time (HTST))	Primary public health safeguard — need to know it has been effective.	Keep pasteurisation records. Check milk with phosphatase test. Reduce contamination by using adequate cleaning and disinfection regimes. Ensure equipment is working properly.
Cool to ≤10°C	If post-pasteurisation contamination occurs, bacteria will grow rapidly if milk stored at higher temperatures.	Cool rapidly.
Refrigerated storage	Possible post pasteurisation contamination.	Clean storage tanks thoroughly.
Filling into bottles or cartons	Bottles and cartons may be contaminated.	Wash bottles thoroughly and keep cartons in hygienic conditions.
Refrigerated storage and transport	Growth of bacterial contaminants.	Keep refrigerated.

General Notes

The Milk (Special Designation) Regulations 1989 require pasteurised milk to be cooled to no more than 10°C. Similar requirements exist in Scotland and Northern Ireland.

Similar considerations apply to the production of pasteurised cream.

ANNEX 5.8

PRODUCTION OF CHEDDAR

PROCESS	PROBLEM	ACTION
Standardisation of cheese milk	Raw milk may be contaminated with pathogens.	Check bacteriological quality of milk.
Pasteurisation (e.g. HTST)	Ineffective pasteurisation will enable survival of pathogens.	Record time/temperature; check efficacy with phosphatase test.
Addition of starter culture	Slow acid development may result in proliferation of other bacteria including pathogens.	Obtain starters from a reliable source and rotate to minimise contamination, check acid development.
Renneting		
Cutting		
Scalding (temperature raised to around 40°C)		
Whey drainage		
Cheddaring		
pH generally reaches 5.2 to 5.3	microbial contamination	Check pH to ensure fermentation proceeding normally, use adequate cleaning regimes, monitor environment and product.
Milling and salting		
Pressing		
Wrapping		
Ripening		

General Notes

1. In some automated systems acid development may be expected to continue in the presses. In such systems the starter should have good salt tolerance as the salt content will not be constant.

2. Pasteurisation of cheese milk is not a universal practice and if raw milk is used good hygienic practice is even more essential. Pasteurisation, however, cannot substitute for good hygienic practices as recontamination can occur.

ANNEX 5.9

PRODUCTION OF SOFT MOULD RIPENED CHEESE (e.g. CAMEMBERT)

PROCESS	PROBLEM	ACTION
Cheese milk standardisation	Raw milk may be contaminated with pathogens.	Check bacteriological quality of milk.
Pasteurisation (e.g. HTST)	Ineffective pasteurisation will enable survival of pathogens.	Record time/temperature; check efficacy with phospatase test.
Addition of starter culture	Slow acid development may result in other bacteria including pathogens proliferating.	Obtain starter culture from a reliable source and rotate to minimise contamination.
Renneting		
Whey removal		
Moulds (shaping of curd)	microbial contamination	Check pH to ensure fermentation proceeding normally, use adequate cleaning regimes. Monitor environment and product.
Salting or brining		
Ripening eg at 12-15°C RH 90-95% 10-14d		
Packed & stored at 4°C		

General Notes

1. Soft mould ripened cheeses develop pH values in excess of 5.0 which may allow any contaminating microorganisms, including listeria, to multiply. For this reason production of soft cheese is of particular concern and particular attention must be paid to hygiene and storage temperatures.

2. Pasteurisation of cheese milk is not a universal practice and if raw milk is used good hygienic practice is even more essential. Pasteurisation, however, cannot substitute for good hygienic practices as recontamination can occur.

Department of Health

PRESS RELEASE

Richmond House
79 Whitehall
London SW1A 2NS

Telephone 071-210 5963

10 February 1989

ADVICE TO THE PUBLIC ON LISTERIA AND FOOD

Sir Donald Acheson, Chief Medical Officer at the Department of Health, today issued general advice to the public about Listeria in food. He also gave specific advice to pregnant women and to some patients, who are particularly vulnerable because of their illness or treatment, to avoid eating certain cheeses.

Sir Donald said:

"Public attention has recently been drawn to findings of the presence of Listeria monocytogenes in a number of different food products. It must be remembered that Listeria is widely distributed in the environment and some exposure to this organism is unavoidable. Indeed at any one time a number of us, perhaps as many as 1 in 20, carry this bacteria in our gut without any ill-effects.

"The disease, listeriosis, caused by infection with this organism is fortunately still quite rare. Last year 287 cases were reported, although it is certain that there were some other unreported cases. When it occurs it can give rise to a mild 'flu-like' illness, although more serious cases may develop meningitis and septicaemia. Of considerable concern is the fact that in pregnant women it may also infect the developing baby and lead to miscarriage, stillbirth or severe illness in the newborn baby.

"Unlike most of the bacteria causing food-related illness that we have been used to dealing with in the past, Listeria has the unusual property of being able to multiply at the sort of temperatures which may be found in refrigerators. Fortunately in most foods where it is present, it occurs at very low levels and is killed by adequate cooking.

"However, for some soft cheeses, the situation is different because the method of preparation and the time they may be kept before eating allows Listeria to multiply. *High numbers* of Listeria have been found in several varieties of soft cheeses, and a number of cases of listeriosis — both in this country and abroad — have been associated with eating heavily contaminated soft cheese.

"Because of this, having taken the best possible expert advice, I would advise that pregnant women should avoid eating certain types of soft cheeses. It is not possible to specify precisely the cheeses in which Listeria is likely to grow, but on the basis of current information these are likely to be soft ripened cheeses such as the brie, camembert, and blue vein types. On the other hand, hard cheeses such as the cheddar and cheshire types, processed cheeses, cottage cheeses and cheese spreads have not given cause for concern.

"The levels of Listeria that have been found in other foods such as cooked-chilled meals and ready-to-eat poultry have usually been very low. Given the particular risks to the developing foetus I feel, however, that it would be prudent for pregnant women to re-heat these types of food until they are piping hot rather than to eat them cold.

"Otherwise, all that is necessary is for pregnant women to follow the normal, general hygiene precautions summarised overleaf and to take care that they maintain a well-balanced diet during their pregnancy.

"Other people who appear to be at special risk and should therefore follow this advice are those with underlying illness which results in impaired resistance to infection, such as patients who have had transplants, those on particular drugs which depress the immune system, and those with leukaemia or cancers of the lymphatic tissues.

"I am sure that the rest of us have become worried about reports of Listeria contamination of a variety of foods, including salads and some of the cooked-chilled ready-to-eat foods on sale. The evidence so far is that the amount of Listeria in these foods is generally very low, and provided that the good hygiene practices I recommend overleaf are followed there is no need for us to change the type of food we regularly eat and enjoy".

GENERAL ADVICE TO THE PUBLIC

Listeria monocytogenes is widely distributed in the environment, for example, it has been found in vegetation, water, soil and the faeces of man and animals and therefore some exposure to this organism is unavoidable. For the average healthy member of the public the risk of becoming ill with listeriosis from eating food is very small indeed. Nevertheless there are a number of simple precautions which the public can take which will reduce their exposures to Listeria and other pathogenic bacteria:—

i. Keep foods for as short a time as possible, follow the storage instructions carefully and observe the 'best-by' and 'eat-by' dates on the label;

ii. Do not eat under-cooked poultry or meat products. Make sure you re-heat cooked chilled meals thoroughly and according to the instructions on the label. Wash salads, fruit and vegetables that will be eaten raw;

iii. Make sure your refrigerator is working properly and is keeping the food stored in it really cold;

iv. Store cooked foods in the refrigerator away from raw foods and cheeses;

v. When re-heating food make sure it is heated until piping hot all the way through and do not re-heat more than once;

vi. When using a microwave oven to cook or re-heat food observe the standing times recommended by the oven manufacturer to ensure that the food attains an even temperature before it is eaten;

vii. Throw away left-over re-heated food. Cooked food which is not to be eaten straight away should be cooled as rapidly as possible and then stored in the refrigerator.

ANNEX 5.11

PRODUCTION OF SKIMMED MILK POWER

PROCESS	PROBLEM	ACTION
Raw Milk	Can be contaminated with pathogens.	Check bacteriological quality of milk product.
Separate	Microbial contamination.	Use adequate cleaning regimes.
Raw skimmed milk	(as above)	
Pre-heat the raw skimmed milk to 80-120°C (depending on the plant used, etc)	Process guarantees microbiological safety and must be carried out properly.	Ensure heat treatment carried out properly — keep time/temperature records etc.
Evaporate at approximately 70°C		
Spray drying		Use adequate cleaning regimes.
Conveying	Microbial contamination	Maintain equipment and keep packaging in hygienic conditions.
Bagging		
Storage		

ANNEX 5.12
PRODUCTION OF STIRRED YOGHURT

PROCESS	PROBLEM	ACTION
Concentrated skimmed milk heat treated (eg 85°C/20 min)	Pathogens may be present.	Ensure heat treatment is carried out, record time/temperature.
Add other ingredients eg sugar syrup, stablisers	Possible contamination from ingredients.	Set specifications for ingredients and monitor quality.
Heat treatment (eg 90°/2 sec)	Destruction of contaminating bacteria to allow growth of culture.	Record time/temperature.
Cool to 40°C and inoculate		
Incubation to suitable pH		Low pH will prevent growth of contaminating organisms.
Cooling		
Mix in fruit conserve, etc	Conserves, purees etc may be contaminated with bacteria and/or yeasts and moulds.	Heat treat to reduce yeast and keep pH of purees etc <4.5 to prevent bacterial growth and toxin production.
Packing	Possible source of contamination.	Keep packaging materials in hygienic conditions.
Cooling		
Refrigerated storage and distribution	Prevent damage to packs	Pack in suitable materials and train staff in handling techniques.

General Notes

1. Equipment should be cleaned after each batch is produced.

ANNEX 5.13

PRODUCTION OF ICE CREAM

PROCESS	PROBLEM	ACTION
Mixing of ingredients including skimmed milk powder, milk fat, sugar	Possible contamination from ingredients.	Set specifications for ingredients and monitor quality.
Pasteurisation	Ineffective pasteurisation will enable survival of pathogens which may be present.	Check efficacy of pasteurisation and its compliance with legal requirements.
Homogenisation	Post-pasteurisation contamination.	Use adequate cleaning regimes.
Cooling & refrigerated storage of mix	Microbial contamination.	Check temperature control.
Freezing of ice cream		
Packaging	Possible source of contamination.	Keep packaging materials in good hygienic conditions.
Hardening and storage		

General Notes

1. Soft serve ice cream presents different problems. The heat treated mix is made up and sold direct from the freezer to the consumer. Inadequate cleaning of equipment can result in product contamination.

ANNEX 5.14

PRODUCTION OF BUTTER

PROCESS	PROBLEM	ACTION
Raw milk	May be contaminated with pathogens.	Check bacteriological quality of milk keep cool and separate from heat treated product.
Separation and pasteurisation of cream	Ineffective pasteurisation will enable survival of pathogens.	Record time/temperature. Check efficacy with phosphatase test.
Cool to <5°C and age		
Butter maker		
Add brine to correct water and salt content (for salted butter)	If emulsion not correctly formed, bacteria present may grow.	Ensure emulsion is correctly formed with small water droplets throughout product, so bacteria cannot grow.

CHAPTER 6

FISH AND SHELLFISH

INTRODUCTION

6.1 The fish and shellfish industry encompasses a wide range of activities, but relatively few of these generate problems of microbiological safety. However, this chapter examines the areas of concern that there are, under the following headings:—

— economic and legislative background (paragraphs 6.2-6.5);

— general fish hygiene (paragraph 6.6);

— scombrotoxic fish poisoning (paragraph 6.7);

— bivalve molluscs (paragraphs 6.8-6.17);

— warm water prawns (paragraphs 6.18-6.20);

— pre-packed smoked fish (paragraphs 6.21-6.28).

BACKGROUND

Economic

6.2 The domestic fishing industry provides about 66% of United Kingdom fresh, chilled and frozen fish supplies by volume. By value, it provides about one third of total UK fish supplies including prepared, preserved and semi-preserved fish. Cod, haddock, whiting, herring, plaice and sole are found in the North Sea; mackerel, together with hake and other demersal fish, off the west coast of Scotland; sole, plaice, cod and whiting in the Irish Sea; and mackerel, sole and plaice off the south-west coast of England. Prawns, crabs, lobsters and other shellfish are found in the inshore waters all around the coast. At the end of 1988 there were about 17,000 fishermen in regular employment and over 5,000 occasionally employed.

6.3 The fish farming industry has seen considerable growth, with production increasing tenfold during the 1980s. By 1989 the wholesale value of farmed fish and shellfish amounted to £140 million. Atlantic salmon and rainbow trout are by far the most commonly farmed, and then oysters and mussels. The industry makes an important contribution to the rural infrastructure, especially in the Highlands and Islands of Scotland.

Legislative

6.4 There are no regulations specifically covering fish and shellfish hygiene in United Kingdom food safety law. In England and Wales, fishery products, like other food items, must satisfy the Food Hygiene (General) Regulations 1970 as amended, and where appropriate, the Imported Food Regulations 1984. Shellfish beds in England are controlled under the Public Health (Shellfish) Regulations 1934 (see paragraph 6.9 below). All these Regulations are administered by the Department of Health. Similar, but separate, provisions apply elsewhere in the United Kingdom. The Fisheries Departments of the Ministry of Agriculture,

Fisheries and Food, the Department of Agriculture for Northern Ireland and the Welsh Office Agriculture Department, are responsible for fisheries policy matters, such as EC negotiations, administering the European Community's Common Fisheries Policy, fisheries research, trade and fish farming.

6.5 As part of the Single Market Programme (see Part II, paragraphs 1.25-1.28), the European Commission has recently proposed a number of measures concerning hygiene standards in the fish industry. Directly relevant are a proposal for a Council Regulation laying down "the health conditions for the production and placing on the market of fishery products" (COM (89)645); and a proposal for a Council Regulation laying down "the health conditions for the production and the placing on the market of live bivalve molluscs" (COM (89)648).

GENERAL FISH HYGIENE

6.6 Fish and shellfish have a range of microbial flora that largely reflects that of their environment. Therefore, unless they are taken from contaminated water, fresh and freshly frozen fish products are generally of high microbiological standard. However, fish and fish products do spoil rapidly and, like other foods, may be subject to cross-contamination. Good manufacturing and handling practices are therefore essential: as in other parts of the food industry, we would stress the vital importance of adopting a Hazard Analysis Critical Control Point approach.

SCOMBROTOXIC FISH POISONING

6.7 One public health problem which can arise if fish is not stored properly is scombrotoxic fish poisoning. This is caused by substances formed by microorganisms growing on the flesh of certain species of oily fish such as mackerel and tuna. The condition is characterised by headaches, rashes and vomiting, and these symptoms can vary considerably in severity. Recovery is usually quite rapid, but on very rare occasions the condition can be fatal. According to data collected by the PHLS Food Hygiene Laboratory (FHL) and the Communicable Disease Surveillance Centre, Colindale (CDSC) there were 42 confirmed incidents of scombrotoxic poisoning in the period 1986-89 and an additional 118 suspected but unconfirmed incidents. There have been no reported fatalities in the UK. Scombrotoxic poisoning can be avoided by ensuring that raw fish used as an ingredient is kept as fresh as possible by storing in ice, by proper refrigeration or by freezing. The precise nature of the substances that cause scombrotoxic fish poisoning is not known, but they are not readily destroyed by heat and the condition is most frequently associated with canned or smoked products. Raised levels of histamine, often found in fish which have caused scombrotoxic fish poisoning, are used as a likely indicator of the presence of causative substances.

BIVALVE MOLLUSCS

6.8 Bivalve molluscs such as mussels, clams, oysters, cockles and scallops feed by filtering the water in which they live. In the process, they can ingest and concentrate bacteria and viruses. Since most bivalve shellfish beds are in estuaries or in inshore waters, they are often close to areas prone to contamination in varying degrees by sewage and other outfalls. Bivalve molluscs may consequently accumulate pathogenic microorganisms at levels which can, when eaten, pose risks to human health. Scallops grow in deep water and so are less subject to this contamination. Relocation of the industry is not feasible, and so it is important that, in areas where contaminants are present, measures be taken to reduce contamination of the end product to a safe level. This is particularly so in the case of oysters, which are eaten raw, where purification is the only control measure.

6.9 The pattern of treatment, which has evolved since the problem of harvesting bivalve molluscs from polluted waters was first recognised in the nineteenth century, comprises "re-laying", "depuration", heat treatment, or a combination of these treatments (see figure 6.1). Re-laying involves relocating the molluscs in

Figure 6.1
STAGES IN THE HARVESTING AND TREATMENT OF BIVALVE MULLUSCS
Oysters, Mussels, Clams

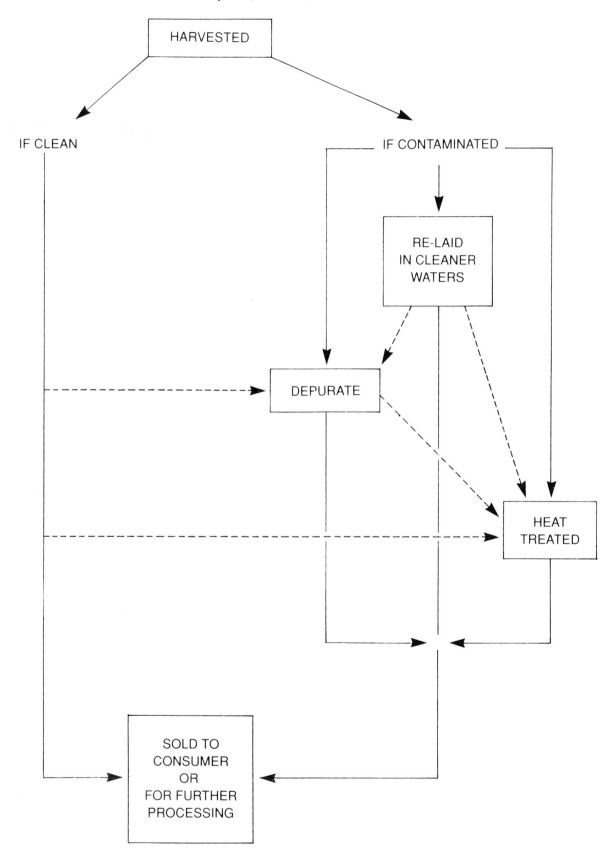

NB: Cockles are normally cooked or
heat-treated before sales to the consumer;
they are not re-laid or depurated.

cleaner waters where they cleanse themselves naturally. Depuration speeds up the process by placing the molluscs in tanks subject to a continous flow of recycling salt water decontaminated, for example, by ultra violet light. Cockles and some mussels are cooked commercially before sale and the heat treatment, if carried out properly, is sufficient to render the product safe. Local authorities have the power to require shellfish harvested from designated areas to be re-laid, depurated or heat treated, under a system of "closure orders" operated under the Public Health (Shellfish) Regulations 1934 (see paragraph 6.4 above). If necessary, the orders can prohibit the lifting of shellfish altogether.

6.10 In practice, most oysters and mussels from England and Wales, even from relatively clean water, are routinely depurated. In Scotland the depuration of shellfish has not up to now been necessary. We are satisfied that depuration is an effective treatment for the removal of bacteria and that is has contributed to the virtual elimination of bacterial diseases hitherto transmitted by molluscs. For example, the last recorded cases of typhoid fever due to molluscs in the UK were in 1958. However, we are concerned that current methods of depuration do not appear to reduce the viruses responsible for hepatitis or for viral gastroenteritis to sufficiently low, non-infective levels.

6.11 Viral contamination of molluscan shellfish has caused numerous incidents of foodborne illness. The principal viruses concerned are hepatitis A and viruses of the Small Round Structured Virus (SRSV) group. These viruses are considered in more detail in Appendix 3 to this second part of our report. Significantly, evidence from documented disease outbreaks has clearly implicated viral agents from shellfish which have been depurated. For example, oysters depurated for 72 hours in a bacteriologically monitored plant caused an outbreak of gastroenteritis in Tower Hamlets during 1983. At least 181 people were affected and SRSVs were seen in the stools of some of the victims. Depurated oysters were also implicated in a gastroenteritis outbreak affecting 71 people in Peterborough in 1984. Depurated mussels were associated with an outbreak of 41 cases of hepatitis in 1979 and depurated English clams exported to America have caused extensive outbreaks of gastroenteritis; at least 14 individual outbreaks involving over 2,000 cases occurred in New Jersey and in New York during a single 3 month period.

6.12 Limited laboratory studies on the effectiveness of the depuration process in eliminating different viruses from molluscan shellfish indicate that some viruses are more easily removed than others. For example, experimentally introduced polio virus can be rapidly and effectively removed whereas hepatitis A virus, although significantly reduced in numbers, may persist at infective levels. We have no knowledge of how successfully the SRSV group are eliminated, because they cannot be grown in the laboratory and there are no methods to detect them in shellfish. Even low numbers of SRSVs and hepatitis A virus are of concern given the likely low infective dose of these organisms.

6.13 In order to develop and evaluate more suitable depuration processes, we identify a need to study the actual viral pathogens of concern, ie those causing gastroenteritis and hepatitis. Methods need to be developed for the detection and enumeration of these viruses. We note that the World Health Organisation (WHO) makes such a recommendation in its Report "WHO Consultation on Public Health Aspects of Seafood-borne Zoonotic Diseases" (WHO/CDS/VPH/90.86, Recommendation 5.7.4). **We recommend that the Government fund research into detection methods for small numbers of SRSVs and for hepatitis 'A' virus in molluscs. We further recommend that this research be followed up to evaluate and, if necessary, to improve the depuration process or to develop new techniques for the elimination of viruses from live bivalve molluscs (R(II)6.1).**

6.14 A substantial reduction in the microbiological pollution of many stretches of inshore coastal waters to a level where depuration is no longer necessary is unlikely in the short or medium term. We believe that the present system of local authority control orders therefore needs to be improved. The European Commission's proposed new Regulation (see paragraph 6.5 above) would classify shellfish growing areas on a systematic basis according to the level of microbiological contamination of the shellfish grown there, and would specify microbiological standards to be met by bivalve molluscs placed on the market for human consumption. It would require bivalve molluscs to be treated by depuration or by re-laying/depuration where these standards could not otherwise be met.

6.15 We note, however, that the EC proposal relies on the use of traditional indicator organisms such as *E.coli*. There is evidence to suggest that this organism is relatively short-lived in marine conditions and may not be a suitable indicator for the viruses of concern. **We recommend to the Government that research is undertaken to establish better indicators of viral contamination of water than *E.coli* and the other bacterial organisms currently used** (R(II)6.2).

6.16 The test of the EC measure, when adopted, will be whether it reduces the microbiological contamination of bivalve molluscs placed on the market and whether it leads to a reduction in human illness associated with the consumption of such products. **We recommend to the Steering Group on the Microbiological Safety of Food that the effectiveness of the proposed EC Regulation COM(89)648 in reducing mollusc contamination and human illness should be monitored in the UK once it has been adopted and that, if the evidence warrants it, the UK Government should press for the requirements of the Regulation to be reviewed** (R(II)6.3).

6.17 Most shellfish, including cockles and mussels, are cooked before eating. An adequate cooking process combined with measures to prevent subsequent recontamination will give a safe product. Recent research in commercial heat processing techniques has led to the development of the "Torry" process which is used at Leigh-on-Sea for the treatment of cockles (the process is outlined in a Department of Health letter to local authorities of 4 November 1987 and in "Specification for Model Cockle Processing Plant, Torry Research Station, Aberdeen, Document TD2106"). The process involves passing the cockles through boiling water on a conveyor belt so that the internal temperature of the meat exceeds 90°C for not less than 90 seconds, conditions that exceed the Central Public Health Laboratory (CPHL) recommendation for the heat treatment of hepatitis A. Since the introduction of the Torry process the CDSC has received no reports of outbreaks of gastroenteritis or hepatitis associated with the consumption of cockles from Leigh-on-Sea. **We recommend that all processors of bivalve molluscs adopt methods that provide an effective heat process and avoid subsequent cross-contamination** (R(II)6.4).

WARM WATER PRAWNS

6.18 During the late 1960s and early 1970s, imported frozen cooked prawns originating from South and South East Asian countries (so-called "warm water prawns" — eg from the genus *Penaeus*) were frequently found to be of poor bacteriological quality. These prawns had been cooked and peeled in the country of origin and the problem appears to have been one of poor hygiene practices leading to recontamination of the prawns after they had been cooked, probably during the hand-peeling process. A study undertaken by researchers of the CPHL revealed that of 2,335 samples of frozen cooked prawns from Malaysia examined in the period 1969-1975, 1.6% were found to contain salmonellae, and that, of 1,310 samples examined in 1972-1975, 9.3% were found to contain *Vibrio parahaemolyticus*. Agreement was reached in 1975 between trade representatives, Port Health Authorities, the PHLS and the Government on microbiological guidelines against which the acceptability of imported frozen cooked prawns could be assessed.

6.19 The microbiological standard of frozen cooked (warm water) prawns imported into the UK (largely via Southampton) during the period 1976-1980 was monitored by PHLS Laboratories. Of approximately 4,000 batches examined, 11.7% failed the requirements of the 1975 Guidelines. Furthermore, 0.2% of the batches were found to contain salmonellae, and the Food Hygiene Laboratory of the CPHL, Colindale frequently found samples positive for *V.parahaemolyticus*.

6.20 Over the last 10 years imports of frozen cooked (warm water) prawns have remained stable (though there has been an increase in the demand for uncooked prawns which are then processed in this country). The monitoring of cooked prawns has continued, and our information is that between 75% and 100% of all consignments are currently tested by Port Health Authorities with rejection rates of between 3% and 5%. Although this rejection rate is still higher than we would wish, introduction of the 1975 guidelines has led to welcome improvements in microbiological standards. **We recommend that Port Health Authorities should continue their testing of imports of frozen cooked (warm water) prawns. We also recommend that importers be reminded that hygiene standards in the processing plants in the countries of origin are an essential ingredient in effective quality control** (R(II)6.5).

PRE-PACKED SMOKED FISH

6.21 The Committee is concerned that pre-packed fish might constitute a botulism hazard, although we should stress that no incidents of botulism have actually been associated with pre-packed smoked fish sold or manufactured in this country. *Clostridium botulinum* occurs naturally in inland, coastal and estuarine waters and may be ingested in small numbers by a wide variety of fish. Product safety is normally ensured by a number of factors: the low incidence of *C.botulinum* in the fish; adequate processing and storage; and a final heat treatment when the fish is cooked for consumption. In the case of pre-packed smoked fish, there is a likelihood that protection from the risk of botulism is less than complete.

6.22 The bottoms of mud-bottomed commercial fish ponds are not well aerated and can accumulate faeces, uneaten feed and dead fish (though the latter should be cleared daily). This can create conditions suitable for the growth of *C.botulinum* which may, in turn, be ingested by the fish. Farmed trout from such ponds have a higher incidence of *C.botulinum* contamination than have fish farmed in concrete raceways or caught from the wild. **We recommend that, when establishing or replacing their facilities, fish farmers should install concrete raceways for the cultivation of trout, instead of mud-bottomed ponds** (R(II)6.6).

6.23 The heat treatment applied during the smoking of fish is not sufficient to destroy *C.botulinum* or its toxin. The factors which effectively prevent growth and the formation of toxin in smoked fish are salt content and temperature. Duration of storage is a factor in control. These factors are particularly important for those smoked fish, such as salmon and trout, which are usually eaten raw. Others, such as kippers and smoked haddock, are normally cooked by the consumer before they are eaten, but this heat treatment may not be sufficient to destroy any toxin present.

6.24 Current demands are for lower levels of salt in many foods, including smoked fish. Thus, products which have not hitherto posed a risk, because their salt concentration prevented the growth of *C.botulinum*, may now do so. The level of salt required varies depending on the temperature at which the product is to be kept, its intended shelf life and the species of fish concerned; smoked trout and mackerel support growth of *C.botulinum* better than other smoked fish. **We recommend that, to prevent the growth of *Clostridium botulinum*, all producers of smoked fish ensure that salt levels are maintained at adequate levels** (R(II)6.7).

6.25 Our concerns are exacerbated by the growing practice of pre-packing smoked fish in modified atmosphere or vacuum packs. The lack of oxygen suppresses normal spoilage, and extends the life of the product by a few days, but it will not prevent the growth of *C.botulinum*, which is an anaerobe. If the organism is present in these products and not adequately controlled by salt levels or by refrigeration, it may produce toxin before the product is appreciably spoiled.

6.26 Strict control of refrigeration and product life is essential for pre-packed smoked fish. Research data accumulated by MAFF scientists at Torry Research Station, Aberdeen, suggests that 3.5% salt in the aqueous phase would be adequate to inhibit toxin production in vacuum packed smoked fish stored at up to 10°C. Nevertheless they advise a storage temperature of less than 4°C and a product life of 5-7 days to ensure a wide safety margin for such salt-containing smoked fish. We also note that the Government produced guidelines on recommended practices for the safe processing, handling, and cooking of fresh, hot-smoked, and frozen trout in 1978. The advice in these guidelines is relevant not only to the industry but also to the small number of consumers who home smoke fish. **We recommend that the Government should update their guidelines on the handling of trout and extend them to other fish species** (R(II)6.8).

6.27 We are particularly concerned at the growing sale of pre-packed smoked fish by mail order — a practice which destroys the integrity of the chill chain. **We recommend that persons should not be allowed to engage in the supplying of smoked fish by mail order unless they are able to demonstrate that their products will not support the growth of pathogenic microorganisms at ambient temperatures** (R(II)6.9).

6.28 We note that the Food Hygiene (Amendment) Regulations 1990 place smoked fish among the products which will be required to be kept at below 5°C unless they have been subjected to processing designed to prevent the growth of pathogenic microorganisms at ambient temperatures. We welcome this as a positive step towards stricter controls on storage temperatures for the products discussed in paragraphs 6.21-6.27 above. In addition, **we recommend that the Regulations which the Government has announced its intention of making on the production, storage and distribution of vacuum packed and other hermetically-sealed products should contain requirements aimed at ensuring the microbiological safety of pre-packed fish, as we understand the Government intends that they should** (R(II)6.10).

CHAPTER 7

TRANSPORT

INTRODUCTION

7.1 Potential microbiolgical problems are associated mainly with food products requiring low temperatures in order to maintain their microbiological integrity. Hence this chapter is primarily concerned with refrigerated transport. Product-specific transport considerations are discussed in the relevant chapters of both parts of our Report. Transport of foods from retail outlets to the home is considered in chapter 10.

7.2 Although a substantial quantity of food imports is still shipped by sea, an increasing proportion, especially from within Europe, is now transported by lorry. Imports by air are restricted to very small qauntities of high value perishable products. Transport of food within the United Kingdom is almost exclusively by road although some food, particularly fish on ice, is carried by rail. The latter presents little microbiological risk provided attention is paid to general cleanliness and hygiene and appropriate precautions are taken in cases of breakdown to ensure that low temperatures are maintained.

7.3 It is estimated that some 300 million tons of food, drink and tobacco, including agricultural products, are transported annually by heavy goods vehicles within the UK with additional volumes carried in smaller vehicles. There has been little growth in the amounts transported in recent years, reflecting the increased efficiency of the food industry with foods transported in processed form, and the major food retailing chains operating centralised warehousing systems.

7.4 There has, however, been considerable growth in refrigerated transport within the UK with the number of refrigerated or insulated heavy goods vehicles increasing by 20% to almost 12,000 over the five year period to 1988. It is estimated that some 20 million tons of food are carried in refrigerated transport and further volumes in insulated lorries. The cost of transporting and distributing food is of the order of £3-4 billion per annum with some two thirds of this accounted for by refrigerated transport.

7.5 There are many different types of vehicle which carry chilled foods. These range from small commercial vehicles relying on insulation to keep pre-chilled foods cool during transport to large heavy goods vehicles with independent cooler units. Most refrigerated vehicles consist of an insulated chamber fitted with a temperature control unit which circulates cool air around the chamber. The chamber may be part of a rigid body or form a trailer with its own chassis and wheels. For long distance transport, especially by sea, the chamber and cooler unit are mounted on a frame and may be loaded for road use onto a carrier trailer or other vehicle.

GENERAL PRINCIPLES

7.6 In order to maintain the microbiological integrity of the food it is as important that adequate attention be paid to hygienic practice during transport as elsewhere. All foodstuffs must be handled and packaged with appropriate attention to their microbiological status. Clear handling instructions should appear on the products to facilitate this, a point to which we return at Part II, paragraph 8.24. The design of vehicles for ease of cleaning and the regular use of microbiologically effective cleaning regimes are also of the utmost importance in all kinds of transport.

7.7 Much transported packaged food (eg canned and dry foods) and bulk food material (eg cereals) is microbiologically stable at ambient temperatures. In such cases careful handling eg stacking is important to avoid damage to packs. Cross-contamination of bulk loads can occur from other parts of the load, from the environment or from a previously carried load. Cleanliness and general hygiene standards are the main factors to which food transporters must direct attention.

LEGISLATION AND CODES OF PRACTICE

7.8 Some consignments of perishable foodstuffs are transported entirely within the United Kingdom; others travel internationally. These categories are covered by separate regulations in the United Kingdom at the present time.

7.9 In Part I, Annex 9.2 we commented on the then proposed amendments to the Food Hygiene Regulations — now the Food Hygiene (Amendment) Regulations 1990. When fully implemented these will set a two-tier requirement for perishable foodstuffs under chilled storage, requiring them to be held at not more than 5°C, or 8°C, depending on risk from pathogens such as *Listeria monocytogenes*, up to and including retail. These conditions will apply to temperature during transport. As noted in our earlier comments there is a derogation allowing small delivery vans to maintain at 8°C for up to 12 hours products for which the prescribed temperature is 5°C. We comment on this further at paragraph 7.19 below.

7.10 Prior to the Food Hygiene (Amendment) Regulations 1990 there were very few statutory hygiene requirements covering purely domestic transport within the UK. There are very basic requirements regarding cleanliness in the Food Hygiene (Market Stalls and Delivery Vehicles) Regulations 1966. The only other existing temperature requirement for domestic food transport is for poultry meat. The Poultry Meat (Hygiene) Regulations 1976 implement EC Directive 71/118/EEC and lay down temperatures for the immersion cooling of carcases, and a maximum temperature for poultry meat in cutting rooms, storage and transport (4°C).

7.11 The Agreement on the International Carriage of Perishable Foodstuffs and on the Special Equipment to be used for such Carriage, commonly known as the ATP (from the French text "Accord Relatif aux Transports Internationaux de Denrées Périssables et aux Engins Spéciaux à Utiliser pour ces Transports"), to which the UK is one of 27 signatory countries, facilitates international traffic in certain perishable foodstuffs for human consumption by setting common and centrally recognised standards. It sets out the warmest temperatures permissible for each of the foodstuffs listed in the ATP; and lays down common standards for the temperature controlled equipment in which these foodstuffs are carried.

7.12 The International Carriage of Perishable Foodstuffs Act 1976 (as amended), and the International Carriage of Perishable Foodstuffs Regulations 1985 make it an offence to permit the use, without good reason, of equipment covered by the terms of the agreement without a certificate of compliance issued by the authorities designated by the Department of Transport. The temperature conditions for the carriage of frozen and chilled products as specified by the ATP are listed in Annex 7.1 to this chapter together with the requirements of the Food Hygiene (Amendment) Regulations 1990 and those of the European Community.

7.13 Within the European Community there has been a great deal of legislative activity in the food hygiene area, especially to secure basic standards for intra-Community trade during the 'lead in' to completion of the single European market (see Part II, paragraphs 1.25-1.28). In addition to the Poultry Meat Directive (see paragraph 7.10 above), specific Directives deal with fresh meat (64/433/EEC), meat products (88/658/EEC), mince and small pieces of meat (88/657/EEC), heat treated milk (85/397/EEC), and egg products (89/437/EEC). Most of these deal *inter alia* with transport.

7.14 Several of the EC Directives lay down temperature controls for specific products (eg poultry meat, fresh meat, meat products, heated milk and egg products). Many of these are currently being updated and additional measures covering other foods are proposed. At present only the Poultry Meat Directive and Egg Products Directive relate to domestic transport and the latter has yet to be implemented in UK law: a statutory consultation exercise on the domestic Regulations implementing the provisions on egg products adopted by the Community so far, including temperature requirements, was initiated by MAFF on 11 June 1990. The other Directives only cover trade between member states, but when updated will apply to all trade within the EC. The requirements of the EC measures, existing and proposed, are similar to those currently required by the ATP and adherence to temperature conditions along the lines of the ATP will therefore soon become necessary for purely domestic transport within the UK.

7.15 Directive 89/108/EEC covers quick frozen foods. It reflects the French concept of a quality distinction between quick frozen and other frozen foods. The underlying principle of the Directive is that foods must be frozen as quickly as practicable, labelled as quick frozen foods and kept at or below −18°C from production through to retail. Practical considerations of temperature maintenance have led to certain temperature tolerances being allowed. Distribution has a 3°C tolerance mainly to allow defrost of equipment. Local distribution has a 6°C tolerance, but this is to be reduced to 3°C in 1997.

7.16 Various bodies produce guidelines for the handling and distribution of chilled and frozen foods. The Institute of Food Science and Technology guidelines for the preparation and handling of chilled foods, recently updated, cover tranport. We are also impressed by the guidelines for handling the distribution of chilled foods, produced jointly by the trade associations 'Tranfrigoroute' and the Cold Storage and Distribution Federation, which deal with the matter in greater detail, particularly in relation to the temperature requirements during storage, loading, transport and unloading. We believe that they provide a sound basis for the hygienic handling of food material. **We recommend that the Government, in collaboration with the relevant industry and professional bodies, should produce a Code of Practice based on existing guidelines, for all transport of refrigerated foodstuffs** (R(II)7.1).

MICROBIOLOGICAL CONSIDERATIONS

7.17 We have, elsewhere in our Report, drawn attention to the important effect of temperature on the rate at which pathogenic microorganisms will grow in foods. We have particularly emphasised the vulnerability of some categories of food and the increasing popularity of such products as cooked chilled foods which require careful temperature control for safe handling and distribution.

7.18 Some pathogenic bacteria, *Listeria monocytogenes*, *Yersinia spp*, and some strains of *Clostridium botulinum* in particular, are capable of growth at temperatures below 5°C. They do not grow rapidly at such low temperatures, but growth can increase sharply as temperatures rise above 5°C. This is an important issue when considering the upper temperature limits that may be accepted throughout the whole of the cold chain. It is particularly so in relation to transport, where temperature control is necessarily more difficult to achieve because of the need to load product onto vehicles and to off-load often at a number of different delivery points.

7.19 We are concerned, as we discussed in Part I, Annex 9.2, that the Food Hygiene (Amendment) Regulations 1990 could permit foodstuffs normally designated as requiring to be held at temperatures not greater than 5°C to be held at 8°C for up to 12 hours during transport in small delivery vans. We understand that a 2°C tolerance is normally allowed on such measurements so that a vulnerable product could be held at temperatures as high as 10°C for prolonged periods; a situation which we consider microbiologically unacceptable. **We recommend that the temperature requirements of the Food Hygiene (Amendment) Regulations 1990 should apply without derogation to all forms of refrigerated and insulated transport, that the Steering Group on the Microbiological Safety of Food should monitor the situation, and that the Government should consider the Food Hygiene (Amendment) Regulations 1990 to be of an interim nature and keep its requirements under careful review (R(II)7.2).**

7.20 Although pathogenic microorganisms may survive in frozen foods they will not grow at the temperatures at which such products are normally held. Upper temperature limits for such materials are determined primarily by quality considerations and there is no microbiological risk when such temperatures are exceeded provided the material remains fully frozen.

OPERATING PRACTICE

7.21 It is important to recognise that the refrigeration equipment used in pre-distribution stores, in refrigerated transport vehicles and for storage of foods in retail and catering establishments, is designed to maintain the temperature of previously chilled products. It is not normally designed to lower the temperature of warm products or of products at ambient temperature. The temperature of foodstuffs during distribution should not be allowed to rise significantly above their storage limit. Excellent temperature control can be achieved, but in practice frequently is not. For effective maintenance of temperature control a refrigerated trailer should be able to reverse up to a properly designed insulating buffer surrounding the loading door in a cold store wall. When the door is opened, the buffer ensures that the connection between store and vehicle is sealed against the ambient temperature.

7.22 The time taken to load or unload a vehicle is an important factor in temperature control; small vehicles capable of rapid handling will require less elaborate arrangements than larger, slower trailers. It can, however, take several hours to load or unload a large trailer, and the proper maintenance of temperature is impossible when this takes place at an unbuffered loading or unloading bay. In the absence of an effective temperature seal during loading and unloading it is necessary to switch off the refrigeration plant on a vehicle in order to prevent rapid condensation of the coolers and subsequent icing problems. Under these conditions it becomes virtually impossible to control temperatures effectively. **We recommend to cold store operators that when new storage and loading facilities are being designed particular attention should be paid to the principles of loading pre-chilled produce into pre-cooled vehicles and adequately protecting the store/vehicle interface from higher ambient temperature (R(II)7.3).**

7.23 There are many designs of refrigerated and insulated vehicles and in general they are capable of maintaining specified temperature conditions provided they are used properly. Particular points needing attention are:—

— products to be loaded should be at the correct temperature;

— the interior of a vehicle should be pre-cooled prior to loading;

— correct operating practice should be followed during loading (eg refrigerated curtain-sided trailers should not be loaded through the side of the vehicle with the curtains drawn back);

— products should be carefully stacked to allow proper air circulation both within the vehicle and during storage at either end of the journey;

— temperature-controlled vehicles compatible with relevant ATP classifications should always be used;

— vehicles should be properly maintained (for example, damage to internal or external panels can allow moisture penetration which can in turn lead to deterioration of the insulation);

— the cleaning regime should include the cooler unit and regular checks that the defrost drains are free from obstruction; overspill from these drains can lead to contamination of product.

7.24 Indirectly monitoring the temperature of the load by measuring and recording air temperatures throughout a journey is an essential part of maintaining control of the cold chain during distribution using refrigerated vehicles. Strategically placed thermometer probes measuring the temperature of cold air reaching the load and that of return air to the cooler will give information about both the efficiency of the chiller unit and the effectiveness of air circulation (packing pattern). Ideally such sensors should be fitted as an integral part of the vehicle and temperatures should be recorded automatically. Chart recorders provide a continous record of temperatures during a journey but it is also important for the driver to have a visual display of temperatures, or an audible warning system activated when temperature control fails. **We recommend to fleet operators that temperature monitoring facilities be fitted to existing vehicles wherever possible and that such facilities should be incorporated in all new refrigerated vehicles** (R(II)7.4).

7.25 Air temperature measurement as described in paragraph 7.24 above is not appropriate for smaller multi-drop delivery vehicles or for simple insulated vans. Here between-pack measurements should be made at the beginning and end of journeys using regularly checked probes.

7.26 Some retailers set strict standards and ensure that these are met, essentially by specifying and monitoring the temperatures of foodstuffs during transport and on receipt. From our observations of distribution operations we are convinced that it is possible to maintain temperatures within closely defined limits during the transport and during loading and off-loading, by the use of suitable equipment and by adhering to well-established operating practices.

CONTROL OF THE TRANSPORT INDUSTRY

7.27 We are aware that the United Kingdom is one of several European countries which have not extended the ATP provisions to purely domestic movements of perishable goods. We believe that the ATP could provide an excellent basis for the establishment of effective legislation controlling the transport of perishable goods within the United Kingdom. Some minor modification to the detail set out in the Agreement may be necessary. We believe that the absence of regulations along these lines in the UK is a serious impediment to the food industry in its attempts to maintain effective temperature control throughout the food supply chain. **We recommend that Government consider the modification of domestic legislation so that the conditions set out in the ATP can be applied to domestic transport as soon as possible** (R(II)7.5).

7.28 Maintenance and certification of vehicles is important. We have been told by trade sources that one of the consequences of the United Kingdom's decision not to apply the ATP domestically is that refrigerated vehicles whose performance has fallen below ATP standards, so that they are no longer certifiable for use in other European countries, are being sold into the UK market where such certification is unnecessary. We understand that the ability to achieve and hold low temperatures declines rapidly in ageing refrigerated vehicles and we are concerned about the possible introduction of such refrigerated vehicles to the UK transport system. It is the industry's responsibility to ensure that the equipment it is using is capable of achieving the temperatures laid down in law. We strongly urge that persons buying and operating second-hand refrigerated vehicles should check the maintenance records thoroughly and satisfy themselves that the equipment is capable of performing effectively.

7.29 We note that EC Directive 89/461/EEC, aimed at harmonising the overall length of articulated vehicles to permit a maximum of 16½ metres, fails to legislate for the design of refrigerated vehicles. Longer vehicles are now being produced. We are concerned that inadequate air circulation in the longer articulated vehicles can lead to inability to control load temperatures effectively. **We recommend that those involved in the design and construction of longer refrigerated vehicles pay particular attention to ensuring adequate temperature control** (R(II)7.6).

TRAINING

7.30 As elsewhere in the food supply chain, the adequate training of staff is essential for the maintenance of hygienic conditions. Temperature integrity can be lost rapidly by poor handling procedures during pre-delivery storage, loading and unloading. The driver of a temperature-controlled vehicle has a particular responsibility for ensuring that the produce being carried is held at the appropriate temperature throughout a journey. **We recommend that all staff handling food during pre-distribution storage, loading and unloading of vehicles, and drivers of refrigerated vehicles, should receive adequate training in the principles of basic food hygiene, temperature control and product protection** (R(II)7.7). We draw attention to the Members' Code of Conduct published by 'Transfrigoroute' which contains an excellent outline of the training requirements for drivers of refrigerated vehicles.

7.31 EC Directive 89/438/EEC, amending 74/561/EEC, lays down the conditions for granting licences to haulage operators. The directives require that operators take an examination of professional competence in a range of topics and the amending Directive adds the carriage of foodstuffs to the list of topics covered. The relevant examination in this country is the Certificate of Professional Competence (CPC) administered by the Royal Society of Arts based on a syllabus established by the Department of Transport. The syllabus of the CPC is currently being extended to incorporate the requirements of 89/438/EEC. **We recommend to Government that knowledge on the carriage and handling of perishable foodstuffs and a basic knowledge of food hygiene be included in the tests for the Certificate of Professional Competence** (R(II)7.8).

7.32 **We also recommend that the principles involved in the operation of refrigerated vehicles should be included in the training of environmental health officers who are responsible for enforcing legislation covering the hygiene conditions of the distribution of foods** (R(II)7.9).

TEMPERATURE/TIME MONITORING

7.33 At numerous places in our Report we have emphasised the importance of temperature control for the maintenance of the microbiolgical integrity of raw materials and food products. It is, of course, impossible to separate temperature and time considerations. Microorganisms grow slowly at refrigeration temperatures, but we have seen that some organisms are capable of growth down to 0°C and grow quite rapidly when the temperature exceeds 5°C. A brief excursion above a maximum temperature limit will have little significance, but prolonged exposure to temperatures above the presecribed maximum can have serious consequences.

7.34 During our study of transport, we surveyed the various systems which are available for indicating the temperature/time history of a product as it passes along the food chain. We have mentioned, in paragraph 7.24 above, the equipment used to monitor the temperature during transport but we believe there is also a need for a simple, inexpensive device which could be used "on pack" to indicate the temperature history of a product.

7.35 Several such indicators are available. Some are effective, particularly where they indicate simply whether a specified temperature has been exceeded. The introduction of the time element is difficult however, and we have not been convinced that any of the simpler monitoring devices currently available are sufficiently reliable or reproducible to be of real value for monitoring the temperature history of packs or loads as they pass along the supply chain. Such systems could however be of value to the consumer. We return to this point in paragraph 10.20 below.

ANNEX 7.1

TEMPERATURE CONDITIONS FOR THE CARRIAGE OF FROZEN AND CHILLED PRODUCTS

LEGISLATION	SCOPE	REQUIREMENTS (maximum temperatures)	
ATP (The International Carriage of Perishable Foodstuffs Act, 1976 and the International Carriage of Perishable Foodstuffs Regulations 1985)	International transport of listed products		
Annex 2	Frozen Foods	Ice Cream	−20°C
		Quick Frozen Foods	−18°C
		Frozen Foods	−12°C
		Butter	−10°C
		Tolerance of 3°C	
Annex 3	Chilled Foods	Red Offal	3°C
		Butter	6°C
		Game	4°C
		Milk for immediate consumption	4°C
		Industrial milk	6°C
		Dairy products	4°C
		Fish, molluscs and crustaceans	on ice
		Meat products	6°C
		Meat	7°C
		Poultry & rabbits	4°C
Food Hygiene (Amendment) Regulations 1990	Listed products	Listed "high risk" products (local delivery in vehicles <7.5 tonnes)	5°C
			8°C
		Listed "low risk" products	8°C
		Tolerance of 2°C	
Poultry meat (Hygiene) Regulations 1976	Poultry meat	Storage and transport	4°C
Directive 89/108/EEC	Quick Frozen Food		−18°C
		Tolerance of 3°C	
		Tolerance of 6°C for local transport until 1997	
Directive 88/657/EEC	Intra-Community trade in mince and meat in small pieces	Chilled	2°C
		Quick frozen	−18°C
		Frozen	−12°C
		Long distance vehicles must be equipped with temp recorders.	
Directive 88/658/EEC replacing 77/89/EEC	Intra-Community trade in meat products	Temp requirements should be clearly labelled and food transported at that temperature.	
Directive 64/433/EEC amended by 83/90/EEC and 85/323/EEC etc	Intra-Community trade in fresh meat	Fresh meat	7°C
		Offal	3°C
		Frozen meat	−12°
Directive 89/437/EEC	Egg Products	Chilled	4°C
		Deep frozen	−18°C
		Frozen	−12°C
		Dehydrated	15°C
Directive 85/397/EEC	Intra-Community trade in heat treated milk	Raw milk	10°C
		Heat treated milk	6°C

CHAPTER 8

RETAILING AND WHOLESALING

8.1 In this chapter we consider the following categories of food retailing: supermarkets and grocers, so-called "open-food retailers" (such as butchers, bakers, fishmongers and delicatessens) which sell unwrapped goods, sales of ice-cream, farm shops, sales from stalls and vehicles, and doorstep deliveries. For convenience we also include here points relating to wholesaling.

8.2 The structure of the food retail sector has undergone large changes in the last twenty years. The number of superstores and large supermarkets has grown considerably; the major companies have opened some 450 superstores in the last five years. The number of traditional small family grocers has fallen significantly. With an increased volume of supplies going direct to retailers, the number of wholesalers has also decreased. According to the Business Statistics Office's Retail Enquiry there were in Great Britain in 1987 about 100,000 food retail outlets (ie those retailers primarily selling food), and a further 50,000 retail outlets selling food as a minor concern. There were also 56,000 off-licences and confectioners, tobacconists and newsagents (CTNs).

8.3 The ten largest retail chains now have about 70% of sales of groceries and provisions and about 50% of all retail sales of food, which altogether amounted to some £40 billion in 1989. The retail cooperative societies, who buy mainly from the Cooperative Wholesale Society, and those small independent retailers who also belong to consortia (the "symbol groups" such as MACE, SPAR and VG) each have roughly 5% of food retail sales.

8.4 Large numbers of people work in food retailing. In 1989 food retailers employed over 600,000 staff and a further 100,000 worked in off-licences and in CTNs. Over half work part-time. The Audit Commission survey found that the average number of people handling food in each premise was about 22 in supermarkets and grocers and about 4 in "open-food retailers". Large supermarkets may have over 50 staff.

Table 8.1 **Number of Food Handlers per Premise**

Type of business	Average	Lower Quartile	Upper Quartile
Supermarkets, Grocers etc.	22.3	3	16
Open food retailers eg butchers	4.1	2	5

Source: Audit Commission survey

The upper and lower quartiles provide an indication of the range of size. For some types of premises the average is inflated by a few large businesses.

8.5 Retailers obtain their supplies from three main sources:—

— by delivery from manufacturers or producers;

— by delivery from wholesalers;

— by collection from cash-and-carries, which supply small independent retailers, or from wholesale markets.

8.6 The major retail companies have vertically integrated management systems. This gives them a high degree of control over such factors as the quality of supplies, distribution, the design of their stores and staff training. The benefits of central purchasing and distribution are also available to the cooperative societies and symbol groups, but these operate with a greater degree of independence from the parent organisation and so there is not the same degree of overall control. The large number of independent retailers are similarly limited in their control over many of the factors affecting food safety. This may be a major reason for the finding in the Audit Commission survey that 11-12% of supermarkets and grocers with fewer than 10 employees presented a significant overall health risk, compared with 5% of those with 10-49 employees and none of those with 50 or more.

8.7 Some foods require extra care, especially if unwrapped, and it is not surprising that the Audit Commission survey recorded a higher health risk at bakers and butchers (Table 8.2).

Table 8.2 **Overall health risk in different categories of retailing**

Type of business	Degree of Overall Health Risk		
	Significant or Imminent	Minor	Negligible
Supermarkets and Hypermarkets	6%	37%	56%
Grocers	11%	40%	49%
Butchers	13%	52%	35%
Bakers	17%	48%	34%
Fishmongers	5%	16%	79%
Other	12%	33%	55%

Source: Audit Commission survey. In some cases (eg fishmongers) the sample was very small.

RETAILING AND FOODBORNE ILLNESS

8.8 The PHLS report summarising information on outbreaks during 1986-1988 (see Part II, paragraph 1.17), reported a total number of 1,562 outbreaks, of which 592 were general outbreaks (that is, not confined to one family). Of the 537 outbreaks for which the location was given, 28 were associated with retail premises; of these, 18 were due to salmonella infections resulting from the sale of contaminated cooked meat products and pies, and 7 were caused by *Staphylococcus aureus*.

8.9 Although the number of outbreaks attributed to retail premises is small, nevertheless food contamination in such premises has the potential to affect substantial numbers of people. Outbreaks of foodborne illness associated with retailing are difficult to detect, because cases are usually widely scattered and are likely to be under-reported (see Part I, paragraphs 3.19-20).

8.10 In Part I, paragraphs 4.29-4.32, we recommended that the Steering Group on the Microbiological Safety of Food should consider the arrangements needed to aid the process of tracing back, so that the producer of the food implicated in an outbreak could be identified as quickly as possible. In addition, it is essential that products can be readily located so that, where necessary, appropriate recall measures can be instituted quickly to remove them from the market. It is in the interests not only of public health but also of manufacturers, wholesalers and retailers to have clear procedures so that the recall of products can be limited to specific batches. The EC Lot marking Directive 89/396 (EEC), which must be implemented into national law by 20 June 1991, provides that the producer, manufacturer, packer or first seller within the EC must apply a mark which will allow identification of the lot from which a specific item has come. This will meet part of our objective. Any further action will have to be taken within the context of EC legislation. **We recommend that the Government should institute discussion with wholesalers and retailers with a view to recording identifying marks for all consignments, so far as is acceptable under EC rules, at all stages as they move through the distribution chain** (R(II)8.1).

8.11 The principles of Hazard Analysis of Critical Control Points (HACCP) are applicable to any food operation and its component parts. This includes storage, distribution and retailing (see Part I, paragraph 7.33 and Appendix 4). To help ensure that the food they offer for sale is microbiologically acceptable, retailers should consider the following:—

a. the microbiological state of supplies and their distribution;

b. storage and stock control;

c. refrigeration and temperature control;

d. design of premises and equipment;

e. staff training and awareness;

f. operating practices.

MICROBIOLOGICAL STATE OF SUPPLIES AND THEIR DISTRIBUTION

8.12 The Food Safety Act 1990 will make important changes in the responsibilities of retailers for checking their supplies. The statutory status of the "warranty" defence is to be removed. A defence of due diligence will apply to all the main offences in the Act. Defendants claiming that the offence was due to someone else will have to show that they have taken all reasonable precautions, and exercised all due diligence, to avoid the commission of the offence by themselves or by a person under their control (ie in general an employee). Retailers will also be able to establish the due diligence defence if they satisfy certain criteria set out in Section 21 of the Food Safety Act 1990.

8.13 These provisions will put a clear onus on retailers to ensure that checks are made on the safety of 'own label' food. They also imply that, even when selling branded goods, retailers will have to be more alert than before to any potential problem. We welcome these changes.

8.14 We would therefore expect retailers to require, wherever possible, that food producers, manufacturers and suppliers use HACCP principles throughout their operations, including on matters such as:—

a. recipe and ingredients;

b. manufacturing details;

c. temperature controls;

d. packaging details;

e. labelling instructions;

f. adequate production records;

g. chemical standards, if appropriate;

h. microbiological standards.

8.15 The major retailers have a great deal of influence over the microbiological state of their supplies and their distribution. They are able to set detailed quality and hygiene specifications, and they often have their own transport fleets and central distribution centres. We believe that such influence has had a positive effect on the quality of foods supplied to retail premises.

8.16 Because of the changes referred to in paragraphs 8.2 and 8.3, the wholesale sector is now mainly in the hands of a few major groups, comprising the wholesalers who deliver (the so-called "delivered" wholesalers) and the large cash-and-carry groups. These large groups use their power to influence operating practices. Most are members of the Federation of Wholesale Distributors whose stated policy is to encourage the highest possible standards among their members. We have been informed that the Federation is developing training schemes on topics such as the proper ways of loading vehicles, checking goods and controlling temperatures. We welcome these moves. **We recommend that the Federation of Wholesale Distributors continues to use its membership to disseminate and to promote high standards of food safety among wholesalers** (R(II)8.2).

8.17 Small independent grocers may not have such control over their supplies as major retailers, but will nevertheless have to check supplies in respect of those matters set out in paragraph 8.14 above, as far as possible.

8.18 There appears to be little publicly available information about small independent cash-and-carry operators or their systems of, for example, stock and temperature control. The Committee has been told that there are many cash-and-carries who are not part of any organisation but who serve considerable numbers of small independent retailers and caterers. **We recommend to Government that further information about small wholesalers and cash-and-carry operators be obtained with a view to assessing whether specific guidance needs to be drawn up for this sector** (R(II)8.3).

STORAGE AND STOCK CONTROL

8.19 Food needs to be stored appropriately and the system of stock control should ensure that all food, both refrigerated and non-refrigerated, moves through storage, display and sale on the basis of "first in, first out". Retailers should be aware of the elapsed and remaining shelf life of their supplies. Careful stock control will eliminate many of the potential hazards in this area.

8.20 Foods can be categorised as follows:—

a. processed foods stored at ambient temperature, such as canned and dry packed foods;

b. raw unprocessed fresh food stored at ambient temperature, such as fruit and vegetables;

c. frozen foods;

d. chilled foods, including raw poultry and meat and cooked and ready-to-eat products.

8.21 In general terms foods in category a. and b. and c. above should present little microbiological risk if retailers take reasonable precautions. Frozen foods must be placed in a freezer, ideally at $-18°C$, on receipt and dry and canned products put in a cool dry store which is well ventilated and protected against vermin and other pests.

8.22 Damaged packaging can affect the microbiological state of a product and sensible handling can avoid this. For example, cans should be handled with care so that they are not dented, with subsequent risk of contamination through damaged seams. Knives for opening cases should be used with care to avoid puncturing the packaging of the product inside. Care should also be taken to ensure that the packaging is adequate; in the case of meat the packaging should be such as to prevent fluids dripping on to other products.

8.23 Food in category d. above is the main area in which a risk of contamination and multiplication of pathogens arises. Raw foods should be stored separately from foods that are ready to eat or that require no further cooking. In addition, chilled and perishable foods need to be handled carefully and kept under appropriate temperature control. Refrigeration is considered in detail in paragraphs 8.26-8.31 below.

8.24 In general we are not convinced that food manufacturers provide as much information as they might to retailers and those transporting food about the storage and handling of their products. The outer packaging, in which food is delivered, could be used to give much more information. For small retailers in particular, it would be helpful if some indication could be given on matters such as the priority for getting the product into cold storage. We understand that some of the large retailers are already exploring colour coding for this purpose. **We recommend that food manufacturers should consider including information on the handling and storage of a product on the outside of its packaging (R(II)8.4).**

8.25 Apart from the labelling advice referred to in paragraph 8.24 there is a need for general guidance on proper storage and stock control for the small retailer. The only practical way in which information such as this can reach the small retailer is through the enforcement authorities. Such guidance could be issued to those applying for registration (see Part II, paragraph 1.30), when this is required under the Food Safety Act 1990. **We recommend that the Government should take the lead in consulting all interested parties and in compiling, for distribution to smaller food retailing businesses, an information pack on appropriate storage of goods and stock control (R(II)8.5).**

REFRIGERATION AND TEMPERATURE CONTROL

8.26 The sale of chilled and frozen foods has become a significant part of the food retailing industry. About 60% of shelf space in supermarkets is devoted to such products. If these foods are not handled correctly in retail establishments, microbiological hazards may be introduced.

8.27 The main principles which retailers should observe are:—

— raw and ready-to-eat food should be stored, displayed and handled separately (see paragraph 8.23);

— sufficient chilled storage should be provided to maintain the correct temperatures for the different classes of chilled food;

— chilled/frozen displays should not be overloaded;

— the temperature of the chill cabinets should be regularly monitored;

— the equipment should be properly maintained and frequently defrosted;

— emergency procedures should be developed to cover breakdowns in the refrigeration system.

8.28 Larger retail premises will have one or more refrigerated stores for holding food before display. The air temperature of such buffer stores should be monitored frequently, to ensure that the foods are being held at the required temperature.

8.29 Where no such buffer storage facilities exist, products should be loaded into display cabinets without delay. Most display cabinets are not designed to lower the temperature of food but merely to hold the temperature; they should therefore be loaded with pre-cooled foods. Microbiological hazards will arise if the temperature of the food has risen in transit beyond a safe level, since it will not be corrected in the display cabinet.

8.30 The Committee has been told that, in the course of the consultation on the Food Hygiene (Amendment) Regulations 1990, it emerged that some refrigeration equipment in current use is not capable of keeping foods at the temperatures necessary for microbiological safety. In addition, the Committee was told that second-hand refrigeration equipment, that may not be able to meet legislative requirements, is being offered for sale. **We recommend that retailers purchasing second-hand refrigeration equipment, should ensure that it is capable of achieving and maintaining the required temperatures** (R(II)8.6).

8.31 In Part I, Annex 9.2, we highlighted the need for guidance on temperature measurement, to contribute to uniformity of action by enforcement authorities. We understand that, following the laying of the Food Hygiene (Amendment) Regulations, the Government intends to issue guidelines on how retailers can ensure they are complying with the Regulations, and also to provide information for environmental health officers who will enforce them. We welcome this initiative. **The Committee recommends that there should be uniform and effective enforcement of the Food Hygiene (Amendment) Regulations 1990, so that temperature control requirements are fully met** (R(II)8.7).

DESIGN OF PREMISES AND EQUIPMENT
Design of Premises

8.32 The premises should be appropriately designed to meet the particular demands of the business. Although design needs will, of course, differ greatly between the large supermarket and the small corner shop, the same important principles apply to all retail premises:—

— there should be sufficient space to allow effective separation of "clean" and "dirty" processes, e.g. handling of raw and cooked food, to avoid cross-contamination;

— the layout should allow for easy access to all areas for effective cleaning and working;

— work surfaces should be impermeable and easy to clean; and the finishes on the floors, ceiling and walls should meet the appropriate hygiene requirements;

— the size of preparation areas should be consistent with the demand for the products being prepared;

— there should be adequate sanitary provision including hand washing facilities for the staff; hand washing facilities should be located close to the area in the premises where raw foods, particularly raw poultry and meats, are handled; they must include the supply of appropriate liquid germicide soap and adequate arrangements for hand drying;

— adequate ventilation should be provided;

— effective and safe pest control measures should be enforced;

— adequate space should be allowed for staff and customers.

8.33 In Chapter 10 we advocate that customers should buy chilled/frozen foods last, to help minimise the rise in temperature between the shop and the home. Ideally, the layout of the retail premises should assist customers to do this, and we would encourage retailers to consider this factor when arranging the layout of new or refurbished premises.

8.34 Well designed layout can contribute greatly to good food hygiene practices. Trade associations have a role to play in providing guidelines. The Government codes of practice for enforcement authorities will encourage authorities to pay attention to layout. In the longer term we understand that, under the Food Safety Act 1990, requirements on the layout of premises could be incorporated in a future revision of the Food Hygiene (General) Regulations 1970.

8.35 All too often non purpose-designed and constructed premises are adapted for food preparation and retail use, without sufficient attention to the possible future expansion of business. Cramped working conditions play a major part in lowering hygiene standards and increasing the risk of food poisoning. We consider that there is a need for standard guidance on good practice for retail businesses. **We recommend that the relevant trade associations should take the initiative in producing detailed guidelines on the design of premises for retail businesses** (R(II)8.8).

8.36 We have already welcomed the Government's proposal to issue central guidance to enforcement authorities on the Regulations made under the Food Safety Act 1990 (Part II, paragraph 1.21(f)). **We recommend that attention should be drawn to the guidelines referred to in R(II)8.8, in the codes of practice to be issued under Section 40 of the Food Safety Act** (R(II)8.9).

8.37 There is a need, in our view, to introduce more stringent requirements related to the layout of retail premises in the Regulations. **We recommend to the Government that general requirements relating to the layout of premises retailing food be included in a future revision of the Food Hygiene (General) Regulations** (R(II)8.10).

Design of Equipment

8.38 In Part I, paragraph 7.26, we stated that the proper design of equipment and its correct installation and operation was highly important in the control of food contamination, and hence in reducing the risks of food poisoning in the food manufacturing industry. The same general principles apply to equipment intended for food retailing and for catering. In Part II, paragraph 9.37, we highlight the need for food safety features, such as cleanability and operational effectiveness, to be considered as an important criteria in the design of equipment. **We recommend the Government to bring together appropriate groups, including the Retail Consortium, to promote discussion between equipment manufacturers and retailers aimed at improving the hygienic design of equipment** (R(II)8.11). A similar recommendation for the catering industry is made in paragraph 9.37.

STAFF TRAINING AND AWARENESS

8.39 At the moment there is no legal requirement for those handling food in food businesses to be trained in food hygiene, although some businesses do provide training for their staff. We have already discussed training in relation to the food manufacturing industry (Part I, paragraphs 7.27-7.30). Many of our comments there apply equally to the retail sector. Our response to the consultation document on the training of food handlers, issued by the Department of Health in December 1989, is at Part II, Annex 11.1.

8.40 To assist customers in safeguarding the microbiological safety of food, we would encourage supermarket managers to see that those staff who help customers to pack purchases into bags should be trained to pack goods in a hygienically satisfactory way, having regard to the particular foods.

8.41 The Committee considers that many of the poor practices in the retail sector, particularly in the smaller businesses, flow from ignorance rather than intention. Many small retailers do not belong to a trade association or other similar body, and do not therefore have ready access to guidance and information to assist them to run their shops more hygienically. Up to now it has been difficult to identify a channel through which these businesses could be reached. This will be resolved, to some degree, by the introduction of the new registration requirements, by which all local authorities will know what retailers there are in their area. The local authority channel could then be used to update such information as necessary. As noted in paragraph 8.25 above, this will be particularly helpful for small retailers. **We recommend to enforcement authorities that registration should be used to provide the retail sector with guidance on the Food Safety Act 1990 and the Food Hygiene Regulations, with information on training requirements and available courses, and with any future relevant guidance and information on statutory requirements and good practices** (R(II)8.12).

OPERATING PRACTICES IN DIFFERENT TYPES OF RETAIL BUSINESS

8.42 Retail businesses such as delicatessens, butchers, fishmongers, bakeries, shops selling ice-cream, farm shops, stalls and vehicles and doorstep deliveries are likely to present greater risks of cross-contamination, because of the types of foods sold. In supermarkets there are potential microbiological risks from self-service of unwrapped products. We now deal with these in turn.

Delicatessens

8.43 Delicatessens sell such foods as cooked meats, fermented meats, soft cheeses and pre-prepared mayonnaise salads which can be potential sources of pathogens. The methods of handling these foods also increase the risk from cross-contamination. It is extremely important to ensure that clear separation is maintained between preparation areas and display. Particular attention must be paid to food handling practices including the maintenance of temperature controls.

8.44 To avoid cross-contamination the following good practices should be observed:—

— separate knives and slicing machines should be used for cooked and uncooked meats;

— separate spoons should be used for each product displayed;

— there should be no topping up of short shelf-life products; fresh supplies should not be put on top of old; when finished, the container should be replaced by a clean container and clean utensils;

— there should be no direct touching of food; plastic gloves, film or tongs should be used;

119

— food should not be placed directly on weighing machines but placed on plastic film or equivalent, when being weighed.

8.45 Most slicing machines are difficult to clean and, if they are used for both raw and ready-to-eat meat products, cross-contamination may occur. The extensive Aberdeen typhoid outbreak in 1964 was exacerbated by failure to clean and disinfect a slicer between use, resulting in the contamination of a number of sliced meats. We understand that the EC Directive 89/392/EEC on food machinery covers equipment used by the retail trade, and we encourage the development of the directive. **We recommend that food equipment manufacturers should look into the possibility of developing more hygienic meat slicers for use by the food industry, and that this aspect should form part of the Government-led discussions referred to in R(II)9.8** (R(II)8.13).

Butchers

8.46 There are some 15,000 retail butchers in the UK, many of whom operate to a high hygienic standard. The main product they sell, fresh raw meat, does not pose a particular microbiological safety problem, as long as it is adequately cooked. However, in the Audit Commission survey one in eight butchers fell into the imminent or significant health risk category. The risk of cross-contamination, both from practices and equipment, seemed to represent a particular problem. We are aware that many butchers are diversifying into cooking and selling cold cooked meats, pies, pasties, sandwiches and cheese.

8.47 In the summer of 1989 eleven reports of salmonella outbreaks associated with cooked meats were received by the Communicable Disease Surveillance Centre, Colindale. These outbreaks resulted in around 1,500 people becoming ill. The contaminated meats were produced by small concerns over half of which were retail butchers. On the basis of reported cases of salmonellosis, a single butcher's operations affected 640 people. There were three deaths (see Part II, paragraph 1.21(i)).

8.48 In-depth analysis of two of these outbreaks revealed considerable ignorance of proper food safety procedures, particularly in relation to the need for proper cooking and the avoidance of cross-contamination. These findings are borne out by the Audit Commission survey which found that, in relation to butchers' premises, the factors most likely to lead to significant or imminent health risk were unhygienic practices and lack of awareness by staff and management of basic food hygiene. We therefore emphasise the need for particular attention to be paid to such premises by enforcement authorities, and for steps to be taken to ensure adequate training of management and staff, with thorough monitoring of hygienic practices.

8.49 Butchers and other small producers, who intend to produce ready-cooked food, should be adequately trained in safe food production and good hygiene practice. The Department of Health and MAFF have jointly provided relevant trade associations and enforcement authorities with a 10-point check list of essential points for butchers undertaking this type of operation (Annex 8.1). In the light of the risk to public health, as demonstrated in the outbreaks described in paragraph 8.47 above, **we reiterate the need for the licensing of those premises carrying out butchery and the processing of meat. In the meantime, in the absence of licensing, although all food premises generally will be registered under the Food Safety Act 1990, we recommend that the enforcement authorities pay particular attention to those retail businesses cooking meat on their premises** (R(II)8.14).

| Bakeries | 8.50 Bakers may also diversify into a wide range of products by selling cold meats, meat pies, sausage rolls and cornish pasties, thus providing opportunities for cross-contamination. Products containing meat should be stored at controlled temperatures in accordance with the Food Hygiene (Amendment) Regulations 1990, and should in any case be stored and displayed separately from other bakery products. |

8.51 Cakes and buns containing cream, whether fresh or artificial, need to be kept refrigerated and handled hygienically. Staphylococcal food poisoning and salmonellosis are well known to follow contamination of cream in cakes and confectionery. Hygienic handling of such products is essential. **We recommend to the trade associations, including the Federation of Bakers and the National Association of Master Bakers, Confectioners and Caterers, that they bring to the attention of their members the need for particularly strict hygienic practices when handling products containing meat or cream (R(II)8.15).**

Fishmongers

8.52 The microbiological safety of fish and shellfish is considered in detail at Part II, Chapter 6. There is no particular problem regarding microbiological risks where the sale of wet fish alone is concerned. However, many fishmongers sell shellfish, eggs, meat and game. In such circumstances we stress the need for fish and shellfish, particularly that consumed without further cooking, to be carefully handled, and to be kept chilled and separated from other items, to reduce the risk of cross-contamination. Smoked fish, particularly if vacuum packed, should also be kept under refrigeration to prevent the growth of *Clostridium botulinum* spores. Under the Food Hygiene (Amendment) Regulations 1990 most smoked fish will be required to be stored at or below 5°C. We welcome the introduction of temperature controls for this product.

Self-service

8.53 The Committee notes the increased sale of unwrapped foods as self-service items in shops and supermarkets. Many of these foods, such as fruit, vegetables and salad ingredients, will be eaten raw. We are concerned that they may be contaminated with pathogenic microorganisms during sorting and choosing by shoppers. There is only limited information concerning the survival of viruses and bacteria and the build-up of contamination on such foods. **The Committee therefore recommends to the Steering Group on the Microbiological Safety of Food that research should be undertaken into the contamination of unpacked foods retailed as self-service items (R(II)8.16).**

Ice Cream

8.54 As we have noted in Part II, paragraph 5.56, ice cream mixes are subject to heat treatment prior to freezing and any hygiene problems arise essentially from the way the product is handled at the point of sale.

8.55 Ice cream sold for immediate consumption can be presented in one of three ways:—

— ice cream prepacked in the factory in individual portions or in larger quantities in tubs;

— ice cream delivered to the points of sale in containers from which it is scooped, or otherwise portioned, into cones or wafers;

— soft ice cream dispensed from special machines.

8.56 Individually packed portions of ice cream are relatively free from microbiological risks, provided that the product is adequately processed. Packaging will protect it from contamination and, of necessity, temperature control of ice cream will be satisfactory.

8.57 Ice cream scooped from containers may be subject to cross-contamination from the scoop. The scoop may remain soiled between use and is invariably kept at ambient temperature. It should therefore be kept between uses in a sterilising solution which is changed frequently. Good personal hygiene of staff is essential.

8.58 Soft ice cream is prepared from a sterilised liquid mix dispensed from specialist machinery. "Thick shakes" served in fast food restaurants use similar equipment. The food contact parts of the machinery are complex and difficult to clean; complete dismantling is necessary in order to clean individual components and, even then, some parts are difficult to disinfect properly. Where the machine is located in a mobile vehicle, the facilities to do this are not always readily at hand. In addition, the liquid mix is normally kept well chilled and control of temperature is important. To help ensure acceptable microbiological quality of the product, the manufacturer's instructions on use of the machine should be followed. The personal hygiene of the operator is also important.

8.59 A recent innovation has been the introduction of "self-pasteurising" machines for dispensing soft ice cream. These undergo a pasteurisation cycle, (usually every night), in which any liquid mix stored in the machine and all food contact parts, are heated to pasteurisation temperatures to eliminate any build-up of contamination.

8.60 The Ice Cream Federation and the Ice Cream Alliance have produced guidelines on the hygienic retailing of ice cream. These were updated in 1989 and have been widely distributed. **We recommend that, when selling ice cream which is not prepacked, retailers follow closely the guidelines produced by the Ice Cream Federation and Ice Cream Alliance** (R(II)8.17).

Farm shops

8.61 With the support of Government, and assisted by grants under the Farm Diversification Grant Scheme, many farms are diversifying into the retail sector by opening shops on the farm as an outlet for their own products, and for food from other sources. It is difficult to assess precisely the size of this sector and its future potential, but the number of such operations is increasing rapidly, especially in tourist areas. Some farm environments may provide many opportunities for cross-contamination, particularly where livestock units are close by. We are concerned that the awareness of those operating shops in such circumstances may not be sufficient to protect the public against potential microbiological hazards. Many farmers also take stand space and sell their products at county and local shows where cold storage may well be inadequate. Overall there appears to be very little guidance available to farmers and others operating such enterprises. **The Committee therefore recommends MAFF and DH to draw up guidelines for those operating farm shops; these could be disseminated by the National Farmers Union and by the enforcement authorities as part of the registration process for food premises** (R(II)8.18).

Sales from stalls and vehicles

8.62 The retail sale of perishable foods, which may present a microbiological risk, often takes place from fixed or mobile stalls and from vehicles. Some vehicles are equipped and operated to a very high standard and, with regard to the particular business conducted, bear comparison with the best of fixed premises. Others are seriously defective in the equipment used and in the manner of their operation.

8.63 Some stalls are located in purpose built markets where the type of structure, services and equipment may differ little from shops. Others are in open spaces always used for trading purposes, or on traditional market areas or individual sites. Where a permanent location is used every day there is a tendency towards better services and facilities than is often the case in less permanent or individual sites.

8.64 The ambience of trading from stalls or vehicles engenders in many customers a relaxed attitude to the standards of hygiene and food safety which they would expect and demand in shops or fixed premises. It is important that customers should come to expect the proper standards for display and sale from stalls and vehicles. It is essential that enforcement authorities do not take a partial or lenient view of this sector of the retail trade. Sometimes storage facilities of stall proprietors are located in a different enforcing authority area from that of the retail stall, and inter-authority liaison is needed to check storage conditions.

8.65 In this context we are reassured to note that the Food Hygiene (Amendment) Regulations 1990 will apply the extended temperature controls not only to retail stores but also to market stalls. Although many factors, including cleanliness, personal hygiene, stock control, integrity of food packs, adequate washing and sanitary facilities are important, one of the most critical factors in maintaining microbiological food safety is, in our view, temperature control. Depending on the foods sold and the arrangements for stock delivery, it may be equally important for temperature control to be thoroughly applied in storage premises, transport to the point of sale and on retail display for sale. **We recommend that enforcement authorities should pay particular attention to sales from stalls and vehicles and should ensure close liaison with other relevant enforcement authorities, so that storage and transport provisions for relevant foods supplied to such businesses are also thoroughly checked** (R(II)8.19).

Doorstep delivery

8.66 Some retailers supply food products directly to the customer through doorstep delivery. The product most commonly delivered in this way is milk, although other dairy products, poultry, eggs, bread and soft drinks are also commonly supplied. An insulated store provides some protection for perishable items but proper temperature control will cease to operate from the start of the delivery round until the time that the customer places the goods in the refrigerator. Also, goods left on the doorstep may attract birds and animals, which may introduce contamination.

8.67 Optimum operation of doorstep delivery services requires speedy and efficient supply of goods by the retailer, and prompt storage of goods by the customer; these factors require particular attention during hot weather. Where prompt storage of the goods is not possible, arrangements should be made between the roundsman and the customer which protect the goods from the sun and the attentions of animals. **We recommend that Government consider with industry the preparation of guidance on how to minimise risk from doorstep deliveries of food and drink, and that this guidance should be included in future versions of their food safety booklet** (R(II)8.20).

ANNEX 8.1

10 POINT PLAN FOR SAFER COOKED MEAT PRODUCTION

PREPARATION

1. Clean and disinfect the raw meat preparation area before you start. This area must be separate from any area in which cooked meat is handled.

(A detergent solution should be used to clean surfaces before they are disinfected. It is important to use the correct disinfectant for surfaces and equipment which will not adversely affect the food, and to use it at the appropriate concentration. For guidance on the use of disinfectants see Point 10.)

Wash your hands before and after handling raw meat.

COOKING

2. To cook meat safely so that Salmonella and Listeria are killed, the <u>centre</u> of the meat must reach a core temperature of at least 70°C for 2 minutes or the equivalent.

3. Make sure your cooking equipment can achieve this consistently.

4. The cooking process must be monitored. You should record the core temperature of at least one item from every cook using a probe thermometer. Wash and disinfect the probe thermometer after each use. Remember to check the accuracy of the thermometer regularly.

COOLING

5. Cool the cooked product as quickly as possible. Bacteria multiply most rapidly between 10-55°C and cooked products should be cooled as quickly as possible through this temperature zone. Remember the smaller the joint the quicker it cools.

6. Store cooked products at 5°C or less in a designated refrigerator.

HANDLING AFTER COOKING

7. Clean and disinfect the cooked product handling area, which must be separate from any area in which raw product is handled.

8. Always wash your hands before handling cooked products.

All equipment must be thoroughly cleaned and disinfected before and after use on cooked foods.

9. NEVER allow raw foods or any other product, used utensil or tool, or surface likely to cause contamination to come into contact with cooked foods.

REMEMBER THAT FOOD POISONING FROM COOKED FOODS OFTEN OCCURS AS A RESULT OF CROSS-CONTAMINATION FROM RAW FOODS.

HELP AVAILABLE

10. Your Trade Associations or your local Environmental Health Officer will be only to pleased to help you if you need any advice on the safe handling of foods, and on disinfectants.

Help and advice on checking that cooking equipment is working properly may be obtained from the Meat and Livestock Commission. (Enquiries to John Goodman telephone number 0908 677577).

EQUIVALENT CORE COOKING TIME/ TEMPERATURE

Temperature	Time
60°C	45 minutes
65°C	10 minutes
70°C	2 minutes
75°C	30 seconds
80°C	6 seconds

CHAPTER 9

CATERING

9.1 Catering is one of the largest industries in the UK. In 1988 the financial turnover for those businesses for whom catering was the main activity was in the order of some £26 billion. The industry has a large number of outlets of very different kinds as shown in Table 9.1:–

Table 9.1 **Catering food premises by type (England and Wales)**

	Estimated number
Hotels and guest houses	35,000
Restaurants, cafes, and canteens	59,000
Pubs, clubs, and bars with food	76,000
Take-aways	24,000
Hospitals	3,000
Educational establishments	25,000
Residental homes	16,000
TOTAL	238,000

Source: IEHO Annual Report 1987-88 and Audit Commission estimates.

We have been told that the total number of catering outlets is not expected to change significantly by 1992, although the number of meals served will probably go up considerably.

9.2 The catering industry largely consists of small independent businesses. The four largest UK national companies represent a turnover of less than 10% of the total. The large number of outlets, their diversity and the absence of any fully representative umbrella organisation makes it difficult to communicate with caterers. There are a number of trade associations but none cover more than a small part of the industry.

9.3 The catering industry is now one of the largest employers in the UK and is the most labour intensive sector of the food industry. In 1987 there were about 2 million catering employees compared with about 0.5 million in 1969. Over 50% of the staff work part-time. Many are agency or temporary staff. Table 9.2 shows the typical numbers of staff in the principal types of outlets.

Table 9.2 **Number of Food Handlers per Premise**

Type of business	Average number	Lower Quartile	Upper Quartile
Hospitals	27.1	6	30
Hotels and guest houses	8.9	2	10
Restaurants, cafes, and canteens	6.4	3	7
Educational establishments	6.0	3	7
Take-aways	5.7	2	5
Pubs, clubs & bars with food	5.4	2	6
Residential homes	4.8	2	5

Source: Audit Commission survey
The upper and lower quartiles provide an indication of the range of size.

9.4 Eating out has increased considerably over recent years and many changes in styles of catering have been developed. The following are some examples of growth areas:—

— the serving of food in pubs;

— hamburger and other fast-food operations;

— "ethnic" restaurants and take-aways;

— pizza parlours;

— roadside restaurants;

— airline catering;

— central production of cook-chill or cook-freeze food, particularly for institutional catering.

While some of these developments may permit improvements in food handling practices, some may introduce new problems for food safety.

CATERING AND FOODBORNE DISEASE

9.5 The Audit Commission survey (Part II, Chapter 1) showed that food hygiene risks in the catering industry varied widely according to the type of establishment. Almost 1 in 5 take-aways and more than 1 in 6 restaurants, cafes and canteens were judged to be a significant health risk, in contrast to fewer than 1 in 7 residential homes and 1 in 20 educational establishments — see Table 9.3.

Table 9.3 **Overall health risk in different categories of catering**

Degree of overall Health risk	Significant or Imminent	Minor	Negligible
Take-aways	19%	47%	34%
Restaurants, cafes and canteens	17%	43%	40%
Hotels and guest houses	13%	40%	46%
Pubs, clubs and bars	11%	45%	44%
Hospitals	7%	34%	59%
Residental homes	6%	37%	57%
Schools and colleges	5%	31%	64%

Source: Audit Commission survey.

9.6 The PHLS/CDSC report (see Part II, paragraph 1.17) gives an analysis of outbreaks reported between 1986 and 1988. Of 1,562 outbreaks of foodborne disease reported, 592 were considered to be general outbreaks (that is, not confined to one family). In 537 of these general outbreaks the location was identified and 438 were associated with the catering industry; of these, 253 outbreaks related specifically to restaurants, hotels and receptions (Table 9.4). Even allowing for ascertainment bias, the figures for catering seem disproportionately high, when best estimates suggest that less than one fifth of the total volume of food passes through the catering sector. It is also noteworthy that, although the general trend has been an increase in outbreaks of foodborne illness, this has not been the case in hospitals.

Table 9.4 **Number of general outbreaks of foodborne disease associated with the catering industry, 1986-88**

Restaurants/Receptions/Hotels	253
Hospitals	80
Institutions	61
Staff Restaurants	27
Schools	17
	438

Note: the location of the other 99 outbreaks was:—
community 18; shops 28; farms 5; infected abroad 26; other 22.
Source PHLS/CDSC report.

9.7 The PHLS/CDSC data showed that the most frequently isolated causal agents in outbreaks from restaurants, hotels and receptions were salmonellas (158) and *Clostridium perfringens* (55). The remainder were caused by *Bacillus cereus*, other *Bacillus spp.* and *Staphylococcus aureus*. The food vehicles responsible were more often detected in outbreaks caused by *C. perfringens, S. aureus* and *B. cereus* than in those caused by salmonellas. The shorter incubation periods in these types of food poisoning probably means that food remnants are more likely to be available for microbiological examination. Poultry (particularly chicken) and other meats were the foods most commonly implicated. The outbreaks due to *B. cereus* were nearly all caused by reheated rice dishes.

9.8 A 1986 report from the PHLS Food Hygiene Laboratory analysed outbreaks reported between 1970 and 1982 and concluded that the single most important factor contributing to food safety problems was preparation of food too far in advance. In general, advance food preparation is more common in catering than in home cooking. In some circumstances it is inevitable: for example, any type of cold meat or food requiring elaborate decoration (gateaux or terrines). On the other hand, food is often prepared in advance for reasons of convenience. The caterer is faced with irregular patterns of trade and peak demands often coincide with unsocial hours. In order to meet these peaks, and to make most effective use of facilities and staff, the caterer will often choose to prepare the food in advance.

9.9 Extended holding of food between preparation and serving presents a danger, since the food may become contaminated and may be stored for too long at unsuitable temperatures. This danger may then be compounded by inadequate reheating. We believe that the training and management of staff should be such that these problems can be avoided by awareness of the following principles:—

— food is prepared in advance only when necessary;

— food is not kept longer than necessary;

— all precautions are taken to avoid contamination of prepared food;

— strict attention is given to cooling food quickly after cooking, and keeping it at the correct temperature;

— food is adequately reheated before serving.

9.10 In Part I, Appendix 4, we described HACCP, a structured approach to the identification of potential hazard points. We acknowledged that, because of the considerable demands made on resources by a full HACCP analysis, it may be inappropriate to a small business with a wide range of different processes, for example catering operations. Nevertheless, **we recommend that caterers should follow a disciplined and carefully structured approach to the identification of** hazards and control points; and that advice to caterers, which we propose in **R(II)9.14**, should emphasise the importance of this approach for the safe management of catering operations (R(II)9.1).

Examples of HACCP analysis of catering processes are given in Annex 9.1.

9.11 Caterers must ensure that all processes under their control are carried out according to the best hygienic practices. We consider these practices under the following headings:—

a. microbiological state of supplies;

b. storage and stock control;

c. refrigeration and temperature control;

d. design of premises and equipment;

e. operating practices;

f. training and staff awareness.

MICROBIOLOGICAL STATE OF SUPPLIES

9.12 Supplies coming into the catering sector fall into three categories:—

i. raw materials, some of which will be cooked before consumption (eg raw meat), while others will have only minimal further processing (eg salad vegetables);

ii. prepared foods which require further handling (eg cooked meats to be sliced, cook-chill dishes to be reheated);

iii. ready to serve foods (eg gateaux).

9.13 Every effort must be made to ensure that supplies meet an acceptable standard of safety. It is the caterers' responsibility to check, as far as is practicable, the source of their supplies, to specify the quality required and to examine such supplies on receipt. Particular attention needs to be paid to foods which can present a higher microbiological risk. A generalised risk categorisation of foods was given in Part I, Annex 7.1.

9.14 Some large catering companies have quality control technologists backed by in-house laboratory services. They pay routine visits to their suppliers to check standards of hygiene. In addition, they may lay down product specifications that are subsequently checked by sampling.

9.15 Most smaller caterers do not have any access to such expertise or laboratory services. Nevertheless, it is important that they seek to satisfy themselves of the microbiological state of their supplies. This is true whether supplies are delivered or whether the caterer collects his food from a cash and carry warehouse. We suggest in Chapter 10 a number of points which the consumer can check in retail shops to identify poor practices. Several of the aspects mentioned are relevant to caterers:—

— delivery vehicles or wholesale premises which look dirty;

— unhygienic behaviour of staff (eg poor food handling, dirty hands, dirty protective clothing, absence of protective clothing, staff who are smoking);

— damaged packaging;

— obviously poor temperature controls;

— lack of separation of cooked and raw foods;

— inadequate date marking or foods which are past their expiry date.

9.16 The storeman, or the person responsible for receiving deliveries or collecting food from the cash and carry, is the first line of defence and should be properly trained to appreciate these points. A systematic procedure should be developed not only to cover general hygiene but also to include specific checks on the temperature of refrigerated foods. If there is any doubt about any hygiene question, the delivery should not be accepted.

9.17 In the Committee's view, smaller caterers need further help in assessing and controlling the microbiological status of their supplies. Enviromental health officers play an important role in ensuring that supplies to caterers are operating to satisfactory standards. **We recommend that, when EHOs inspect premises used for the sale and distribution of food to caterers, they should pay particular attention to the hygienic quality of the products and their storage and transport** (R(II)9.2).

9.18 Food labelling is a related issue. Food sold to caterers must comply with the Food Labelling Regulations 1984. These require, amongst other details, instructions for use and date marking appropriate to the particular food. However, in the case of supplies to caterers, the Regulations allow the information to be provided in trade documents, furnished on or before the delivery of the food, rather than on the food packaging itself. This practice can lead to confusion. Additionally we have been told that supplies to caterers are often inadequately labelled in contravention of the Regulations.

9.19 Amendments to EC food labelling requirements, set out in EC Directive 89/395/EEC will, however, require the name of the food, the name and address of the supplier, an indication of minimum durability (eg "best before" or "use by" date) and any necessary storage conditions, to be given on the external packaging even if they are also given in trade documents. It is proposed to implement these changes in UK law from 1 January 1991. The Committee welcomes the new provisions as they will assist stock control and alert food handlers to the conditions under which food should be kept.

STORAGE AND STOCK CONTROL

9.20 The general principles of good storage are:—

— adequate storage space should be provided;

— foods should be stored at appropriate temperatures;

— a designated store room should be equipped with racks which allow easy access for cleaning;

— raw and cooked food should be separated;

— storage space should be regularly maintained and kept free from pests;

— systematic stock control and stock rotation should be carried out.

9.21 The Committee emphasises the importance of adequate and suitable storage space in catering establishments, although recognising the difficulties in maintaining satisfactory conditions in many premises where space is at a premium. **We recommend that the guidelines for the catering industry referred to in R(II)9.14 should include more detailed advice on storage** (R(II)9.3).

REFRIGERATION AND TEMPERATURE CONTROL

9.22 Poor temperature control has frequently been shown as a cause of food safety problems in catering. The Audit Commission Survey showed that lack of effective monitoring of temperature was one of the five factors recorded most frequently as a high health risk. The caterer should take care to apply appropriate temperature control to all stages of cold holding, cooking, hot holding and re-heating.

9.23 The cooking process is important in killing pathogenic microorganisms. Cooking processes should therefore be checked to ensure that the required temperatures are being reached. Such checks are particularly important for large pieces of meat where the core temperature of the item being cooked may be difficult to establish. Accurate probe thermometers are needed to check the temperature of food during cooking.

9.24 In order to interpret such temperature checks, caterers will also need clear guidance on temperature targets in specific areas, particularly the temperatures for effective cooking of different types of meat. **We recommend that the guidelines referred to in R(II)9.14 should contain advice on the times and temperatures needed for effective cooking of different types of food** (R(II)9.4).

9.25 After delivery, food which needs refrigeration must be put into chilled or frozen store immediately. Any hot food to be stored in the refrigerator should be cooled as quickly as possible beforehand. Cooling should be carried out in a controlled manner using blast chillers, if possible.

9.26 Raw foods requiring refrigeration (eg raw meat and poultry, vegetables) must be kept separate from cooked and ready to eat foods (eg cooked meats, dairy products). Wherever possible caterers should store this type of food in separate refrigerators or cold stores. Frozen raw meat and fish should be fully, but carefully, defrosted before use, avoiding the spread of contamination from "drip".

9.27 Caterers should develop routine procedures for monitoring the temperature of refrigeration equipment daily and for checking that all equipment is functioning properly. Indeed such procedures are implicit in the temperature provisions of the Food Hygiene (Amendment) Regulations 1990. **We recommend that the guidelines referred to in R(II)9.14 should include advice on the maintenance of all equipment and the methods for monitoring the temperature of refrigeration equipment** (R(II)9.5).

DESIGN OF PREMISES AND OF EQUIPMENT

Design of premises

9.28 We commented in Part I, paragraphs 7.20-7.26, on the importance of the design of premises and equipment for the safe manufacture of food. This is equally important for catering. Good design of food preparation areas depends on two distinct aspects. First, the construction materials and finishes must be of a high standard to be durable, to be easily cleaned and to deny access by, or harbourage of, pests. These features have been a general requirement of the Food Hygiene Regulations for many years. Secondly, the size and layout of the kitchen should encourage good product flow and the separation of clean and dirty processes, to reduce the risk of cross-contamination. Many food factories are able to provide almost total separation of cooked and raw food. This is often difficult in a caterer's kitchen, but we believe that better separation through good basic layout and production flow provides the opportunity to control food safety hazards. **We recommend that caterers, when planning a kitchen, should consider the need to provide separate areas for clean and dirty processes, and have regard to good production flow, to reduce the risks from cross-contamination** (R(II)9.6).

9.29 Many catering premises, particularly in urban areas, have to be accommodated within existing buildings. This factor frequently imposes restraints on space and layout. Lack of space and high intensity use can exacerbate the problems of maintenance, cross-contamination, temperature control, cleaning, storage, and pest control. Because of such constraints it is particularly important that the principles of good design and layout are implemented, as far as is possible, from the outset.

9.30 In modern units the design requirements have become more exacting. For example, the increasing use of cook-chill catering has led to the development of higher standards, particularly in the central production unit. Hygiene criteria, acceptable in the early 1980s, need modification to meet the standards specified in the 1989 update of the Department of Health guidelines on cook-chill and cook-freeze catering systems, or the code of good practice for airline catering recently published by the Airline Caterers Technical Co-ordinating Committee.

9.31 The Audit Commission noted in their survey that lack of adequate hand washing facilities was one of the commonest high risk factors in food premises. There should always be adequate sanitary provision, with hand washing facilities for the staff as required by the Food Hygiene (General) Regulations 1970. Ideally hand washing facilities should also be located close to the area in the premises where raw foods, particularly raw poultry and meats, are handled. Hand washing facilities must include the supply of liquid germicidal soap and adequate arrangements for hand drying.

9.32 The Department of Education and Science has issued advice on school meal kitchens and the Department of Health has published a Building Note on the design of hospital kitchens (HMSO ISBN 0113210264). Some local authorities have also issued guidelines on the design of kitchens for catering purposes. We consider, however, that more broadly based and centrally agreed guidance is needed and would be particularly useful for the small catering businesses. Such guidance would do much to improve the standards adopted in new premises and, over a period of time, would improve the standards of existing premises. **We recommend that the guidelines referred to in R(II)9.14 should include advice on the design of kitchens which would be appropriate for catering businesses especially the small independent caterers; and that these guidelines should be used by environmental health departments in offering advice and guidance to such businesses** (R(II)9.7).

Design of equipment

9.33 The design of equipment is equally important. Over the last 10 years the introduction of new types of purpose-built equipment to carry out the basic cooking, refrigeration and reheating processes has mainly affected the medium and large catering operations. By contrast, many small businesses still use equipment designed for domestic use which may not be suitable for commercial operation.

9.34 We agree with the concerns expressed recently about the use of domestic microwave ovens for catering purposes. A recent survey by EHOs found that about half the ovens used by caterers were domestic models. Sustained use of a domestic microwave oven can lead to a build up of heat in the magnetron, which results in a significant reduction in power output. Many models of catering oven include a fan cooling system on the magnetron, which should allow them to operate under conditions of sustained use.

9.35 The Committee are aware that MAFF has asked the Institution of Environmental Health Officers (IEHO) to encourage the use of catering ovens, rather than domestic models, in commercial premises, and has written to organisations in the catering industry on similar lines. We welcome this initiative.

9.36 Although tests were completed in early 1990 on the variability of performance of domestic microwave ovens, there is little information publicly available on the performance of microwave ovens designed for caterers. The Committee is pleased to note that research commissioned by MAFF into the variability of performance of microwave ovens for catering is now in progress.

9.37 Many criteria need to be borne in mind in the design of catering equipment and some of these may make conflicting demands. For example, a compromise may be made on the quality of construction materials (eg aluminium or stainless steel) for reasons of cost. Safety features such as guards may present problems for effective cleaning. We consider that features which may affect food safety must be considered as important criteria in the design of catering equipment. Too often standards are set for electrical and mechanical safety, but do not take account of features such as cleanability and operational effectiveness. We understand that initiatives on European food equipment standards are currently being considered in response to EC Directive 89/392/EEC and that these will apply to all food machinery including catering equipment. A UK response is being prepared by the British Standards Institute. **We recommend that the Government brings together appropriate Groups to promote discussion between UK producers and users of catering equipment, aimed at improving the hygienic design of equipment and, in particular, at ensuring that appropriate EC design standards are agreed upon (R(II)9.8).**

Design of premises and equipment — other considerations

9.38 The Government proposes to use powers in the Food Safety Act 1990 to require new food businesses (including caterers) to register with the local authority at least four weeks before opening. This will provide a useful opportunity for the local authority to give information on operating practices. We believe, however, that four weeks gives little time for any major design problems to be corrected — and we comment on this later in the chapter. **We therefore recommend that anyone intending to open a catering business should contact their local environmental health department as early as possible, and certainly before expensive decisions on layout are taken, so that appropriate information and guidance can be provided** (R(II)9.9). Such arrangements should benefit both the owners of the business and the local authority, by ensuring that the resources of the environmental health departments are directed to identifying and preventing problems rather than reacting to problems after they have occurred.

9.39 Health Authorities are required to involve EHOs in the design of NHS hospital kitchens. The design and equipment of other catering premises are often examined, not only when detailed planning permission is sought, but also when application is made for a liquor licence. The majority of catering premises now require liquor licences, and many local authorities liaise with Licensing Justices to ensure compliance with Food Hygiene Regulations and other relevant legislation, before a liquor licence is granted, renewed or substantially amended. We note that the liquor licensing system in Scotland requires formal certification that (a) planning conditions, (b) building control regulations and (c) food hygiene requirements are met before a liquor licence is granted. All three bear upon the hygienic operation of the premises. Although much good has come from the informal liaison between local authorities and licensing justices in England and Wales, the situation would, in our view, be usefully improved by the adoption of formal certification as used in Scotland. **We recommend that environmental health**

departments of local authorities should be informed and involved whenever planning permission is sought for catering premises or applications made for change of use (R(II)9.10).

9.40 Catering establishments must maintain a clean environment. Surfaces, preparation areas and equipment must be frequently and thoroughly cleaned. Where necessary, equipment should also be disinfected. Equipment which is particularly complicated in design, such as slicers, mincers, and soft ice-cream machines, must be carefully and completely dismantled to allow proper cleaning and disinfection after use. Automatic dishwashers which use very hot water, strong detergent, and air drying should be used whenever possible. For manual 'pot wash', the hottest possible water should be used with a good detergent. The water should be changed frequently. If items are to be dried by hand, disposable towels should be used.

9.41 Cleaning materials are another area where domestic products are not necessarily suitable for commercial use. A number of specialist companies provide a range of chemicals to perform the various cleaning tasks in a catering operation. Suppliers will usually provide back up advice and information on choosing the correct product for each job, and on the safe and effective use of each product. They may even provide more general advice on drawing up detailed cleaning schedules to ensure that all parts of the operation, and all pieces of equipment, are cleaned at the proper frequency, using an appropriate method. Caterers should have a systematic cleaning schedule to ensure effective cleaning of the kitchen and kitchen equipment.

OPERATING PRACTICES

9.42 The organisation of any commercial kitchen depends upon a number of factors. The type and volume of business will determine whether the food is produced by one person or by a full "kitchen brigade" of chefs. In addition, many catering operations are based on styles of cuisine which are relatively new to the United Kingdom. There appears to be a significant increase in the use of ready prepared dishes to replace the cooking of basic raw materials in the catering outlet. These developments provide the opportunity to reduce some potential food safety risks but also introduce some new ones.

9.43 The risks from fast food take-aways producing fish and chips or hamburgers are likely to be low when the food is properly cooked immediately before serving. But other "take-aways", such as sandwich bars, may present a greater risk when food is prepared in advance and there is inadequate temperature control. Cook-chill food may have the advantage of preparation in carefully controlled factory conditions; but the onus is still on the caterer to exercise good temperature control in storage and reheating. Sous-vide technology has the potential to allow growth of *C.botulinum* spores unless both production and storage are carefully controlled.

9.44 Good operating practices are particularly important, because poor or inadequately understood standards are likely to slip under pressure when, for example, business is brisk or during staff shortages. Many sections of the food industry have produced codes of best operating practice but we know of only a few examples in the catering industry where there are similar codes or guidelines. These relate mostly to fairly narrow specialist areas:—

— cook-chill and cook-freeze catering (Department of Health);

— airline catering (Airline Caterers Technical Co-ordinating Committee);

— drinks vending machines (Automatic Vending Association of Britain);

— sous-vide catering (Sous-Vide Advisory Committee);

— outdoor event catering (The Mobile and Outside Caterers Association of Great Britain).

We are also aware of a number of codes produced by individual environmental health departments or by catering companies.

9.45 Throughout both parts of our Report we have recognised the valuable part played by trade associations and similar bodies in the context of food safety. Such organisations can prepare and disseminate useful codes of practice and notes of guidance for their particular sector of the industry. They also serve as a channel of communication between Government and the trade.

9.46 Of all the sectors of the food industry that have concerned us, the catering sector seems the least provided with an umbrella organisation. There are various bodies covering parts of the sector, but none can claim comprehensive coverage and a large membership. In its own interest we believe the industry should take the lead in putting the missing arrangements into place. This would help to remedy what we feel to be a serious lack of guidance and help in relation to food safety. Ideally, we would see these bodies as playing a major role in producing and promulgating a common standard, which could promote best hygiene practice in the catering industry.

9.47 In the meantime use should be made of existing guidance. The Department of Health has published a health service catering manual "Hygiene" (HMSO ISBN 0113210957) for the use of NHS caterers. The manual covers, in considerable detail, hygiene management, food handling, cleaning and maintenance (including design and equipment) and pest control. We understand the Department will be revising the manual as a result of the Food Hygiene (Amendment) Regulations 1990 and of changes resulting from the Food Safety Act 1990. We endorse this initiative. **We recommend that, for the time being, the catering industry and local authorities should use the manual "Hygiene" as a basis to improve standards throughout the industry** (R(II)9.11).

TRAINING AND STAFF AWARENESS

9.48 We have already noted the fourfold increase over the last twenty years in the number of catering employees, and the high number of unskilled staff, agency staff and casuals. As the Audit Commission survey shows, there is a clear link between poor training and health risks – see Figure 9.1.

9.49 The training of catering staff is a complex task of which hygiene training is only a part. Traditionally, the catering industry has used the City and Guilds of London as a recognised source of "craft" training, which has included hygiene training. The larger catering organisations have also developed their own training programmes for all types of staff. There are numerous other sources which caterers may use for staff training; courses are offered by local colleges of further education, local environmental health departments, the Hotel and Catering Training Company and private consultancies. Hygiene training may be the entire course content or it may be simply a module in a broader syllabus. In our response to the Government's consultation document on hygiene training for food handlers, we pointed out the need for a system to ensure uniformity of standards between these various bodies, if the courses are to satisfy a mandatory training requirement.

9.50 We also emphasised that management is responsible for food hygiene and that supervisors with direct line responsibililty should be adequately trained before more junior staff. Good management and supervision is particularly important in

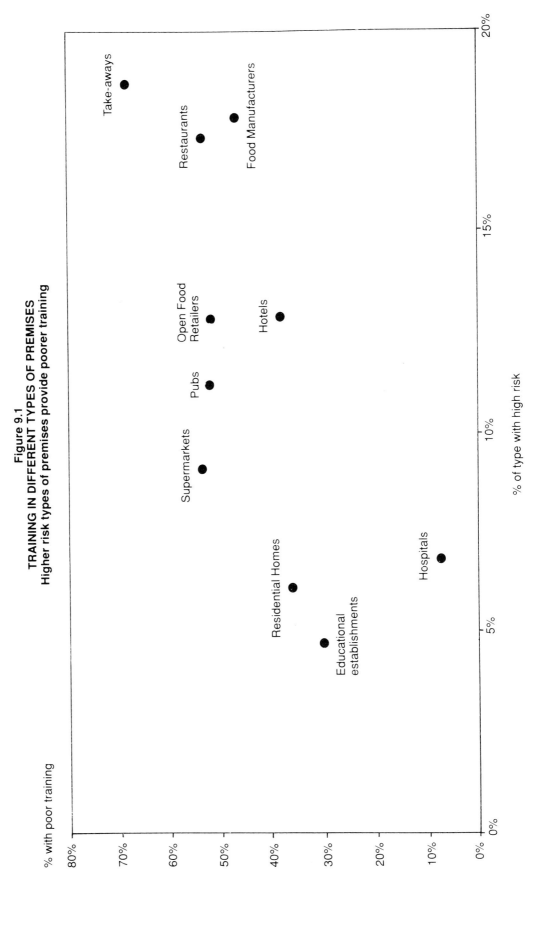

Figure 9.1
TRAINING IN DIFFERENT TYPES OF PREMISES
Higher risk types of premises provide poorer training

% with poor training

% of type with high risk

Source: Audit Commission Survey

136

catering where there is a high turnover of staff and many part-time or casual workers. The basic six hour course on food hygiene would, if taken by all catering staff, have a greatly beneficial effect on current standards. The need for more specialised food hygiene training would depend on the complexity and size of the business.

9.51 The Committee is of the view that proper training and retraining, and continued observance of the principles and practice of food hygiene, are of the greatest importance in reducing food hazards in all catering establishments. Our views are set out in greater detail in our response to the Government's consultation document on the training of food handlers (see Part II, Annex 11.1).

9.52 The Department of Health has produced a booklet "Clean Food" for use in training NHS catering staff. This booklet is available from HMSO (ISBN 011321264X) and we commend it as suitable to be used in catering establishments for in-house training and refresher training.

ENFORCEMENT

9.53 Very many catering outlets operate as small independent businesses with one branch or maybe a few branches in a locality. In common with other small businesses in the food industry, some of which were described in Part I, Chapter 8, these enterprises are unlikely to have technical expertise within the company or to have access to research associations, professional bodies or trade associations who might provide some help. Frequently advice on food safety comes only from the local authority EHO. Although the regulatory function is of vital importance, we think that the environmental health departments should not neglect their role as a source of advice and information.

9.54 At present if standards are unsatisfactory, enforcement authorities have to choose between informal warnings of no legal standing and prosecution in the courts, the only sanction recognised under the law. The system of improvement notices, under the Food Safety Act 1990, will overcome this problem by the introduction of a formal notice whereby managements will be given details of deficiencies and a reasonable time to put things right. The service of such notices is, however, discretionary. While in no way denigrating or wishing to curtail the advisory and educational work done by enforcement authorities, we consider that the use of the formal notice route should be the rule rather than the exception, whenever specific breaches of relevant regulations are found. **We recommend that the Government should incorporate advice on the use of formal notices in the codes of practice for enforcement authorities** (R(II)9.12).

9.55 In Part I, paragraph 9.15, we recommended the development of a new cadre of specialist food technicians to assist EHOs and to enable enforcement authorities to achieve more adequate levels of monitoring. It has also been suggested that better enforcement results can be obtained if there is specialisation, ie with certain environmental health staff concentrating on food premises or commercial premises, rather than carrying out the full range of environmental health duties. A specialist organisation may be suitable for cities and other urban areas where greater concentrations of catering premises occur. It is less likely to be practical in more dispersed areas, where for reasons of travel time and cost effectiveness a generalist organisation will often be more appropriate. In the view of the Committee, such organisational aspects should be addressed by the enforcement authority in the light of local circumstances, eg number, type and dispersal of catering premises and the current staffing levels. We do, however, consider it essential that all enforcement authorities should adopt a system of risk assessment of catering premises in their area, on which a structured approach to monitoring and enforcement may be based. The issue of national codes of practice could help towards desirable conformity across the many enforcement authorities.

9.56 Use of such risk assessment should lead to inspections of premises of sufficient frequency and in sufficient depth to ensure that, not only deficiencies in premises, but also faults in working practices or in management control are identified and steps taken to remedy them. **We recommend that all enforcement authorities should institute risk assessment as a basis for proper monitoring and enforcement. We further recommend to the Government that guidelines on risk assessment be drawn up and issued to enforcement authorities** (R(II)9.13).

9.57 We understand that the Implementation Advisory Committee will be discussing codes of practice relating to hygiene inspections in catering premises and to food standards inspections, including the frequency of sampling. We have already commented in Part I and elsewhere in Part II on the need for greater uniformity of practice among enforcement officers. Many catering organisations that fall within more than one local authority boundary consider that the inconsistency of enforcement of the Food Hygiene Regulations by EHOs, makes their own operational practices difficult to standardise. We therefore strongly endorse the Government's initiative in promoting more consistent standards of enforcement across the country.

9.58 The registration procedures, which the Government has announced it will introduce under the Food Safety Act 1990, will provide an opportunity for local authorities to have some up-to-date information about the number and types of catering premises in their areas. Registration should provide a channel for promulgating information and advice to caterers. **We recommend that the Government should take the lead in drawing up guidelines for the catering industry which include:—**

a. identification of hazard points and control

b. good storage practices

c. temperatures for the effective cooking of food

d. maintenance of equipment and methods of monitoring the temperature of refrigeration equipment

e. design and planning of kitchens including provision of separate areas for clean and dirty processes

as discussed elsewhere in this chapter, and that the enforcement authorities should then consider how to ensure that these guidelines reach individual caterers (R(II)9.14).

9.59 In part I, paragraph 9.9 and recommendation 9.1, we made clear our view that a system of formal licensing involving prior inspection should in due course be extended to all catering establishments. The Audit Coimmission survey reinforces the Committee's view that something more than registration of catering establishments is necessary. **The Committee recommends that the Government should move to the licensing of all catering establishments, as soon as possible** (R(II)9.15).

RESEARCH AND SURVEILLANCE

9.60 There is relatively little research and surveillance carried out on microbiological safety in catering. Local authorities and other bodies have carried out surveys of end products (eg cook-chill food in hospital, sandwiches sold in sandwich bars, and airline meals) but guidance on hygienic practice is usually based upon general microbiological principles rather than on specific research in the catering context. We believe that surveys of catering practice on ways of improving the microbiological status of the end product would be useful. **We recommend that both the Steering Group and the Advisory Committee on the Microbiological Safety of Food should consider further studies on catering** (R(II)9.16).

HOSPITAL CATERING

9.61 We drew attention in paragraph 9.6 above to the fact that, contrary to the trend in the wider community, the number of foodborne outbreaks in hospitals has not risen. The Department of Health attributes this development to a number of factors of which the most important are: commitment to improve food safety on the part of the central Department, individual health authorities (particularly at local level), the hospital control of infection teams and catering managers; a high level of training of all staff handling food; modernisation of kitchens; close liaison with and inspections by environmental health officers; and the lifting of Crown Immunity in 1987. This encouraging experience indicates in our view that it is possible for a large and scattered organisation without any commercial incentive and with staff and buildings of a very diverse nature, to make considerable strides in improving food safety by close attention to better practices and monitoring.

ANNEX 9.1

EXAMPLES OF THE HAZARD ANALYSIS AND CRITICAL CONTROL POINT SYSTEM APPLIED TO CATERING PROCESSES

Example 1

HAMBURGERS

These are typically produced on a cook-to-order basis or with a very short hot holding period.

STEP	IMPORTANCE	HAZARDS	PREVENTATIVE MEASURE (CONTROL)	MONITORING
1. **Raw materials**	CCP	Foodborne illness-causing bacteria in ingredients.	Purchase good quality beef patties from reputable supplier. Proper storage conditions. Stock control.	Check deliveries for quality and temperature. Temperature of storage units.
2. **Raw material storage**		Failure to control may lead to significant growth.	Hygienic design of equipment and preparation area. Effective cleaning and disinfection. Control of temperature. Controlled thawing if to be defrosted before cooking. Control of time and temperature of thawed patties.	Visual check on effectiveness of cleaning. Temperature of storage units. Time of storage of perishable materials.
3. **Cooking**	CCP	Survival of infectious foodborne illness-causing microorganisms if cooking inadequate.	Efficient well maintained cooking equipment. Well established cooking procedure capable of achieving a minimum food temperature in excess of 70°C for 2 mins.	Check temperature of cooking equipment correctly set. Check food temperature where practicable.
4. **Post cook handling and hot holding**		Recontamination with foodborne illness-causing bacteria. Bacterial proliferation.	Hygienic design of equipment and utensils. Effective cleaning of same. Personal hygiene of staff. Cleanliness of garnishes. Minimise hot holding period. Hot holding must maintain food temperature above 63°C. Clean, hygienic packaging material.	Visual monitoring of cleaning. Check staff hygiene. Check hot holding temperature.

140

Example 2

COLD CHICKEN FOR SALAD

Microbiological safety of this product depends on effective cooking of a raw material which is likely to be contaminated with Foodborne illness causing bacteria (especially Salmonella and Campylobacter). Subsequent handling of the cooked carcase when it is portioned must not allow recontamination and effective chilled temperature control must be maintained after cooking until display for sale.

Absolute segregation of raw and cooked processes presents practical difficulties. Monitoring systems used in factories may not be used in a restraurant kitchen where automatic controls may not be available. Display of open foods for customer self-service is rarely found outside of catering operations and may present risks of contamination.

STEP	IMPORTANCE	HAZARDS	PREVENTATIVE MEASURE (CONTROL)	MONITORING
1. Product raw materials	CCP	Foodborne illness — causing bacteria in ingredients.	Purchasing specifications for raw materials. Design of storage facilities and specification of storage conditions. Stock control.	Compliance with specifications. Time (and temperature) of storage of raw materials. Hygiene of storage areas.
2. Raw material preparation		Failure to control preparation procedures may lead to significant microbial growth.	Hygienic design of preparation equipment and preparation area. Cleaning and disinfection schedules for equipment and area. Time and temperature control of perishable materials. Controlled thawing of raw, frozen ingredients.	Hygiene of equipment. Hygiene practices of operatives. Times, temperatures and conditions for holding products during preparation. Storage of prepared materials.
3. Cooking	CCP	Survival of infectious foodborne illness — causing bacteria if cooking is not properly controlled. Prevention of contaminated post-cooking.	Design of cooking equipment including ability to control cooking temperature; cleanability. Use of a cooking procedure that ensures that all ingredients receive a minimum heat treatment 2 minutes at 70°C or an equivalent thermal process. Separation of cooked and raw processes. Protection of product from contamination post-cooking. Cleaning and disinfection of surfaces after their use for preparation of raw food and before their use for cooked foods.	Check cooking procedure (time and temperature). Hygiene of cooking vessels and other containers. Staff and equipment movements.
4. Cooling	CCP	Contamination and growth of microorganisms.	Hygienic design of chiller. Adequacy of cooling capacity. Specification of cooling rate (to prevent growth of microorganisms surviving cooking) and exit temperature of product from chiller. Protection of product from contamination during cooling. Cleaning and maintenance of chiller.	Check product cooling rates and performance of chiller. Hygiene of chiller.

Example 2

COLD CHICKEN FOR SALAD (cont)

STEP	IMPORTANCE	HAZARDS	PREVENTATIVE MEASURE (CONTROL)	MONITORING
5. Portioning the carcass*	CCP	Contamination with foodborne illness-causing bacteria. Microbial proliferation.	Hygienic design of portioning area and equipment. Effective cleaning. Good personal hygiene. Effective separation from 'dirty' processes*. Minimising time product kept above chilled temperature. Chilled ambient conditions if possible. Staff training.	Visual monitoring of cleanliness. Check product temperature. Check practices, especially effectiveness of separation from raw processes. Visual check of personal hygiene standards.
6. Storage	CCP	Microbial growth.	Adequate chilled storage capacity. Capable of achieving 5°C or colder. Stock control.	Check temperature of product and storage unit. Visual check on cleanliness.
7. Display and service	CCP	Microbial growth and contamination with foodborne-illness causing bacteria.	Hygienic design of display equipment. Effective cleaning of display equipment. Temperature control. Control of display period. Packaging, or design of display unit, appropriate to minimise contamination (especially in self-service situation). Provision of suitable and sufficient clean serving utensils.	Check serving utensils available. Replace with clean ones periodically. Check temperature.

*NB A segregated "High Risk" area with separate equipment and dedicated staff is described in Chapter 7 of PART 1.
The opportunity for such an area rarely exists in a multi-use catering kitchen.

Example 3

SLICED MEAT

This example describes the supply of bulk-pack pre-cooked meat from a manufacturer which is subsequently sliced by the caterer for serving cold.

STEP	IMPORTANCE	HAZARDS	PREVENTATIVE MEASURE (CONTROL)	MONITORING
1. Supply of bulk cooked meat	CCP*	Foodborne illness-causing bacteria in the meat when supplied.	Purchase from reputable suppliers. Distribution under effective temperature control. Properly date marked. Where practicable, detailed product specification.	Where possible detailed supplier audit. Where possible check compliance with specification. Check temperature on delivery. Check properly date-marked, and sufficient "life" remaining. Visual check on cleanliness of delivery vehicle ie personnel, and properly packaged.
2. Storage	CCP	Microbial growth.	Effective chilled stores at 5°C or colder. Good stock control.	Check storage temperature. Check stock rotation.
3. Slicing	CCP	Contamination with foodborne illness-causing bacteria. Microbial growth.	Hygienic design of preparation area and equipment (especially slicer). Effective cleaning (especially slicer). Good personal hygiene. Effective separation from 'dirty' processes. Minimum time product kept above chilled temperature. Chilled ambient conditions if possible. Staff training.	Visual monitoring of cleanliness. Check product temperature. Check practices especially effectiveness of separation from raw process. Visual check of personal hygiene standards.
4. Storage	CCP	Microbial growth.	Adequate chilled storage capacity. Capable of achieving 5°C or colder. Stock control.	Check temperature of product and storage unit. Visual check on cleanliness.
5. Display and service	CCP	Microbial growth and contamination with foodborne illness-causing bacteria.	Hygienic design of display equipment. Effective cleaning of display equipment. Temperature control. Control of display period. Packaging, or design of display unit, appropriate to minimise contamination (especially in self-service situation). Provision of suitable and sufficient clean serving utensils.	Check serving utensils available. Replace with clean ones periodically. Check temperature.

*In this example the microbiological safety of the material supplied is of vital importance to the ultimate safety of the food when eaten. Subsequent CCP's may increase the risk but no CCP in the control of the caterer can reduce the level of microbial contamination. Effectively, control resides with the manufacturer and not the caterer.

CHAPTER 10

THE CONSUMER AND THE HOME

INTRODUCTION

10.1 Over the past few decades there have been many changes in the way people shop and buy food, and in the way food is manufactured and sold. These changes have made new and different demands on people using the domestic kitchen to prepare meals. Most food consumed in the UK is prepared in the home from purchased ingredients and is generally eaten without any ill effects. Nevertheless, the incidence of foodborne illness attributable to "family" cases, (that is, those involving only members of the same family), gives cause for concern.

10.2 Domestic kitchens come in different shapes and sizes. In general the kitchen is thought of as a specially designed separate room used by a single family. Some kitchens are, however, converted rooms and from a food safety viewpoint not well designed. They may be shared, for example in student accommodation; or may consist only of a cooking corner in a living or bedsit room.

THE HOME AND FOODBORNE DISEASE

10.3 The PHLS/CDSC report (see Part II, paragraph 1.17) recorded 970 family outbreaks out of a total of 1,562 outbreaks of foodborne illness reported in the calendar years 1986, 1987 and 1988. The annual numbers were almost the same for each year; 326, 324 and 320 respectively. The numbers due to *Salmonella enteritidis,* however, more than doubled from 76 in 1986 to 165 in 1988, being matched with a reduction in other salmonellas. There were a few outbreaks due to other organisms, *C. perfringens* (7), *Staphylococcus aureus* (4) and *Bacillus cereus* and other *Bacillus spp* (13). Family outbreaks have probably been substantially under-reported. In 1989 when computerisation of laboratory data made it easier to link together apparent sporadic cases with the same surname, the number of recorded family outbreaks increased (see Part I, Appendix 1, paragraph A1.22). Nevertheless, family outbreaks are still probably substantially under-reported.

10.4 Although some of these family outbreaks were probably caused by food prepared outside the home, many could be caused by poor hygiene in domestic kitchens. One of the main concerns is the direct or indirect cross-contamination of cooked products by raw products, combined with poor storage. There is a lot of dispersed information on the microbiology of the kitchen which would benefit from being co-ordinated. **We recommend that the Steering Group on the Microbiological Safety of Food should review the available information on the microbiology of the kitchen, and assess the need for further studies of the causes of contamination** (R(II)10.1).

10.5 Bringing contaminated food into the kitchen presents hazards, not only because of microorganisms in the food itself but because of possible cross-contamination of other foods. We emphasise, as elsewhere in the Report, that the greatest care should be taken at all stages of the production and distribution chain to keep food as free as possible from microorganisms capable of causing illness. The kitchen, however, represents the last line of defence in the food chain.

10.6 Provision of microbiologically safe food in the home requires:—

a. supplies of the best possible microbiological state;

b. careful transport home;

c. appropriate storage and refrigeration;

d. appropriate cooking and re-heating methods;

e. adequate guidance on labels;

f. sensible design of the kitchen and of kitchen equipment;

g. effective cleaning;

h. exclusion of pets from food preparation areas as far as possible;

i. hygienic waste disposal;

j. information for the consumer;

k. special precautions for particularly vulnerable groups.

MICROBIOLOGICAL STATE OF SUPPLIES

10.7 The consumer has the right to expect that food on sale will be of the best possible microbiological state. The purchaser should check for poor practices at the point of sale, such as:—

— shops and equipment which look dirty;

— unhygienic staff behaviour (eg poor food handling, smoking, dirty hands, no hand washing between touching raw and cooked foods);

— damaged packaging;

— chilled/frozen displays which are filled above the loadline;

— obviously poor temperature control;

— displays where cooked and raw foods are not separated (eg meats in butchers shops or delicatessens);

— foods which are past their datemark.

We note that the Government information leaflet "Food Safety: A Guide from HM Government" draws the attention of consumers to some of these points.

10.8 If consumers are concerned about any of these points, they should take them up immediately with the store management. Withdrawal of a customer's business can be a powerful incentive to corrective action especially in the case of smaller stores. Uncorrected bad practice should be reported to the Environmental Health Department of the local authority.

10.9 There are also a number of positive steps, which consumers should ensure are taken in the store, to help maintain the safety of the food purchased:—

— raw meat and poultry should be wrapped separately from one another and from all other foods;

— raw foods should be packed separately from cooked goods;

— chilled/frozen foods should be bought last;

— packages of chilled/frozen foods should be packed together; preferably in a cool bag or failing that, in an ordinary carrier bag. (This will minimise the rise in temperatures).

TRANSPORT TO THE HOME

10.10 Because it breaks the "cold chain", transport of food to the home can increase food poisoning risks especially for chilled foods. Recent surveys commissioned by MAFF and the Consumers' Association indicate that approximately 70-80% of consumers take such products home within one hour. However, a small number of consumers take considerably longer, sometimes upwards of three hours. A limited experiment commissioned by MAFF at the Institute of Food Research, Bristol, has shown that chilled food placed in the boot of a car can soon reach very warm temperatures at which food poisoning organisms can multiply rapidly. In the same experiment foods kept in a pre-cooled insulated box remained significantly cooler. However, the public seem largely unaware of the advantages offered by such insulated containers: according to a Consumers' Association survey only 4% claim to use them. **We therefore recommend that chilled foods should be transported home quickly, and that much wider use should be made of cool bags/boxes** (R(II)10.2).

STORAGE AND REFRIGERATION

10.11 Recent consumer advice leaflets and videos (see Annex 10.1) have given useful general guidance on the safe storage of food:—

— once home, chilled/frozen foods should be stored quickly;

— storage instructions on packets should be followed closely, and the packets used in date order and always within recommended dates;

— if there is any doubt as to its safety, food should be discarded;

— all storage facilities, including refrigerators and freezers, should be kept clean;

— care should be taken not to allow cross-contamination between raw and cooked foods, particularly in the refrigerator;

— raw meat and poultry should not be allowed to drip on to other foods.

10.12 Many foods need to be stored by the consumer at low temperature to prevent the multiplication of microbes. The composition of some apparently traditional foods has altered over the years to meet changing tastes. Levels of salt, sugar, smoke and other preservatives have often been reduced. Foods that did not previously need refrigeration may now be highly perishable. These changes make it essential for the consumer to follow the instructions on the pack about storage.

10.13 Although over 95% of households in Great Britain now have refrigerators (General Household Survey 1987), the increased use of longer life prepared foods, eg chilled recipe dishes, has placed much greater demands on domestic refrigerators to ensure the safety of food. In addition, with advances in the microbiological knowledge of pathogens which multiply at low temperatures, the temperatures now considered necessary are lower than those thought acceptable only a few years ago. We believe that changes in the technology of food production have not been matched by corresponding advances in the design of most domestic refrigerators. They are not designed to cool food rapidly and some may not be able to keep it at a temperature which best provides for its safety.

10.14 Most refrigerators have only one chilled compartment. This is commonly used for a variety of foods, some of which are kept chilled to extend their storage life (eg salads, vegetables), some for safety (eg cooked meats) and some simply for convenience or taste (eg butter, drinks). The result is that the temperature of the refrigerator tends to be a compromise between these various needs.

10.15 A number of foods refrigerated for "taste", which are not chilled during distribution and retail display, may introduce a significant heat load when placed in the refrigerator. This is particularly so when large volumes of liquid are involved. The frequent opening of the refrigerator door also makes it difficult to keep the temperature low.

10.16 The design of domestic refrigerators rarely includes forced air circulation and there can be considerable variation in temperatures at different places within the refrigerator. Nevertheless, thermometers can be a useful indicator of the operational effectiveness of a refrigerator. **We recommend that, if their refrigerators do not have a built-in thermometer, consumers should buy a reliable thermometer and use it to monitor the temperature of the refrigerator** (R(II)10.3).

10.17 Some domestic refrigerators coming on to the market offer three or four separate compartments operating at different temperatures. Some of these refrigerators incorporate fan-assisted air circulation, and internal doors which isolate each zone so that opening the door of one compartment does not affect the temperature in other parts of the refrigerator. At present these refrigerators are relatively costly, and the Committee recognises the difficulty in creating a market for significantly more expensive appliances. Nevertheless, **we recommend that the design of domestic refrigerators should include such food safety features as more precise temperature control, separated internal compartments (including a zone at 3°C), and built-in thermometers with external displays** (R(II)10.4).

10.18 To use the existing types of refrigerator most effectively the consumer should:—

— not leave the door open unnecessarily;

— not overload the refrigerator, especially with foods that do not need to be there;

— ensure there is enough refrigerator space to meet the household's needs;

— ensure appliances are regularly defrosted in accordance with manufacturers' instructions;

— if there is no built-in thermometer, buy a refrigerator thermometer to check that the temperature is low enough. Identify the warmest spot in the refrigerator and check the temperature there — ideally the maximum should not exceed 5°C;

— cool hot food before putting it in the refrigerator.

10.19 In Part I we stated that it was of great importance for the safe handling of food that refrigerators should be capable of achieving and maintaining microbiologically satisfactory chill temperatures, and we expressed our concern that the provisons which encourage this in the European Community are currently being weakened rather than strengthened. We reiterate our recommendation in Part I, paragraph 9.8, about the adoption in EC law of requirements on the effectiveness of refrigerators.

10.20 We have noted in Part II, paragraphs 7.35-7.37, that "on-pack" indicators which can monitor either the temperature or time/temperature of a food package as it passes along the chain, are currently being developed. Clearly, an effective, inexpensive system which is easy to operate and interpret, would be of considerable value to the consumer. It would, for instance, enable a consumer to check the temperature history of a product at the point of sale, and to monitor subsequent storage conditions after purchase. We therefore welcome the research project recently commissioned by MAFF, in collaboration with the National Consumer Council, into consumer attitudes to these devices and the problems which could arise in their interpretation. In addition **we recommend that the Government should, in collaboration with industry, sponsor research into the development of a simple, inexpensive and reliable temperature history indicator** (R(II)10.5).

Freezers

10.21 In most households freezers are now the main long-term method of storing perishable foods. It is advisable:—

— not to re-freeze food once it has been thawed;

— to monitor that the temperature is correct, ie less than $-18°C$;

— to defrost the freezer regularly;

— to observe manufacturers' storage instructions;

— to use older products first.

COOKING AND REHEATING

10.22 The application of sufficient heat to food destroys microorganisms. Heating must be sufficient to ensure that a temperature of 70°C throughout the food for at least two minutes (or a time/temperature combination of equivalent lethality), is achieved. This will destroy any level of salmonella, listeria, campylobacter or other none spore-forming organism likely to be found in food. It is immaterial whether the heat is applied by conventional or microwave ovens. Food manufacturers, oven manufactureres and retailers should thus ensure that operating instructions for ovens and instructions on food packs are designed to enable the consumer to cook or reheat the food safely.

Microwave ovens

10.23 Growth in the use of microwave ovens has been rapid and in 1989 nearly 50% of all UK households possessed one. For a whole range of cooking and reheating processes microwave ovens are perfectly satisfactory and they play an important part in many people's lifestyle. Some people are, however, not as accustomed to them as to conventional cookers. Certain characteristics of the microwave oven require the consumer to take greater care than with conventional ovens:—

— microwave ovens are designed to heat in a shorter cooking time and, thus, the margin for error and the opportunity for heat to be transferred by conduction are less than in conventional cooking;

— heating can be affected by different features both of the food and of the oven. This leads to variations in temperature throughout the food.

10.24 Models of microwave oven vary in a number of ways. Whilst total uniformity is neither necessary nor desirable, the present degree of variation gives rise to uncertainty among consumers about performance and use. The Committee welcomes the initiative taken by MAFF in the last year and a half to encourage all concerned — oven manufacturers, the food industry, retailers and consumers — to explore together ways of overcoming this problem, and we welcome the advice already issued on simplifying power ratings.

10.25 The power of microwave ovens, measured in watts, varies to some extent according to the size and type of load being heated. The power rating of an oven will therefore vary, depending on the method used to assess it. As a result, the declared wattages of different models have not in the past all been determined on a comparable basis. This has in turn created a problem in that consumers will have assumed, quite wrongly, that they can rely on cooking or reheating instructions given in recipe books or on food packs being for a microwave oven with the same power output as their own. Food manufacturers have also faced problems devising reliable instructions, given that actual power output can vary markedly among ovens of the same declared output. The Committee therefore welcomes the agreement by members of the Association of Manufacturers of Domestic Electrical Applicances (AMDEA) to adopt from September 1990 a standard method of determining declared power output in ovens, based on the International Electrotechnical Commission (IEC) standard 705. We also welcome the extension of this agreement on a voluntary basis to those manufacturers and importers who are not AMDEA members. The Committee believes that, to avoid uncertainty and confusion, it is highly desirable for all microwave ovens sold in this country to be rated to the same standard. **We therefore recommend that all manufacturers of microwave ovens should adopt a standard based on the IEC standard 705, for assessing the power rating of ovens marketed in the UK** (R(II)10.6). We note with approval that the European Community is working towards a Europe-wide standard. We also understand that work is currently being carried out to refine this standard and expand its application internationally.

10.26 As explained above, from a food safety point of view the value of a uniform method of determining the power rating of ovens lies in the user being able to match this rating to heating instructions. It follows that consumers need to be able readily to establish the power rating of their oven. **We therefore recommend that all manufacturers of microwave ovens should label the front of the oven conspicuously with an indication of its power rating assessed in accordance with the IEC standard 705. We further recommend that manufacturers should display simple operating instructions conspicuously on the front of microwave ovens, on the lines of many other types of domestic appliances** (R(II)10.7).

10.27 It is important that the operating instructions for the oven and the cooking instructions on the packets of prepared food should be compatible. We welcome the agreement between MAFF and members of the Microwave Working Party that "as soon as practicable instructions on microwavable (sic) foods will be appropriate to ovens rated accordingly to IEC 705".

10.28 A wide range of power ratings complicates the food manufacturers' task of providing clear labelling information. We welcome the proposal that five power ratings should be adopted. We hope that this will be implemented as soon as possible.

10.29 It is important that owners of microwave ovens produced before the IEC standard is adopted should be able to discover their oven's rating according to the agreed standard. **We recommend that microwave oven manufacturers should inform owners of models produced before the IEC standard is adopted, of their oven's rating according to that standard** (R(II)10.8).

10.30 Standardisation of power rating, however, will not deal with variation in the evenness of heating within any particular oven. Research commissioned by MAFF and carried out by the Institute of Food Research has shown that significantly different temperatures may be obtained in different parts of the oven cavity. Racks, turntables and wave stirrers have been produced by various manufacturers to try to overcome the problem of unevenness in heating but we are not convinced that these provide a wholly satisfactory solution to the problem. **We recommend that microwave oven manufacturers should carry out more research to evaluate properly which design features most affect unevenness of heating, and should pay attention to the need for evenness of heating when designing new models** (R(II)10.9).

10.31 When cooking raw food, care should be taken to follow the instructions of the microwave oven manufacturers. Carrying out instructions about stirring, turning and standing time should help to ensure the microbiological safety of food.

10.32 The characteristics of any food product affect its suitability for microwave heating. Where food manufacturers put instructions for microwave heating on food labels they should ensure that the food will be microbiologically safe after heating by this method.

10.33 There is, however, some confusion among consumers about which prepared dishes are suitable for microwave heating and which are not. We consider that:—

— if a food is suitable for microwave heating the instructions on the pack should say so;

— if a food is definitely unsuitable for microwave heating eg because it could be damaged, this should be stated.

We recommend that a code of practice should be developed jointly by food manufacturers and microwave oven manufacturers, to determine a basis for establishing microwave heating instructions (R(II)10.10).

10.34 **We recommend that the manufacturers of microwave ovens should ensure that clear guidance on those foods which are suitable for microwave cooking, and those which are not, is included in the recipe books they usually supply with their equipment** (R(II)10.11).

10.35 If there are no instructions on the label, then the consumer should assume that the product is not suitable for microwave heating and the instructions for conventional cooking should be followed.

Pre-preparation/Cooling

10.36 Particular care should be taken in handling food which is prepared some time in advance of consumption eg for home entertaining. An analysis of 1,479 general and family outbreaks of foodborne infection reported to the Public Health Laboratory Service between 1970 and 1982, (see paragraph 9.8 above) showed that the most common contributory factor was preparation too far in advance of needs (57%), followed by storage at ambient temperature (38%) and inadequate cooling (30%). Where two or more of these factors are present, then the risk to the microbiological safety of a food item is greatly increased. In cases of bacterial food poisoning, one or more factors may cause the initial contamination in a food item to become an infectious or intoxicating dose. The initial dose of organisms in a food is usually insufficient to cause food poisoning, but the presence of sufficient nutrients, moisture and warmth, together with a time lapse before consumption, may allow the microorganisms to reach harmful levels.

10.37 Food prepared for eating at some later date should be rapidly cooled and, if possible, then stored in a refrigerator. Pre-prepared food should not be left unrefrigerated for longer than necessary and should, certainly, be stored in a cool place. If prepared food is to be transported to the place of consumption the use of a cool box is highly recommended. Re-heating food after it has already been cooked is a potentially hazardous process. Particular care should be taken to ensure that the food is thoroughly reheated right through to the centre. No food should be reheated more than once.

Barbecues

10.38 Considerable microbiological risks may be associated with barbecues, particularly because of the nature of the cooking process, the handling practices and the exposure to environmental contamination. To minimise such risks the following precautions should be taken:—

— the food awaiting cooking should be kept cool;

— the meat/poultry should be checked to ensure that it is cooked throughout;

— after cooking, the food should be held at a hot enough temperature (eg at least 63°C);

— cooked and uncooked foods should be kept separate to avoid cross-contamination;

— all foods should be covered to avoid contamination by flies, dust, fumes etc.

LABELLING

10.39 Labelling provides an important source of information for consumers about the food they buy. On microbiological safety the consumer requires information in three areas:—

— Durability Regulations based on EC Directive 79/112/EEC require "best before" or "sell by" dates to be shown on most foods. Under Directive 89/395/EEC "sell by" dates will be phased out by 1993 and "use by" dates introduced for foods which are "highly perishable and are therefore likely after a short period to constitute an immediate danger to health". We welcome the Government announcement that, for perishable foods, "use by" dates will be required from 1 January 1991 when "sell by" dates will also be phased out. This is in line with the recommendation in Part I (paragraph 9.25).

— Storage The Food Labelling Regulations 1984 require information on storage to be included on the label of foods where necessary, eg "keep refrigerated". Such labels also often have a considerable amount of other information, both required and voluntary. We consider that in negotiating and implementing new statutory initiatives, the Government should ensure that the prominence of important messages on microbiological safety should be maintained.

— Instructions for Use The Food Labelling Regulations 1984 also require pre-packed food to be labelled with 'instructions for use' in certain circumstances. Most manufacturers and retailers do provide good instructions for use of their products, including cooking or reheating procedures, and often refer to more than one method. We welcome this. We make specific reference to instructions relating to microwave heating in paragraphs 10.24-10.35 above.

KITCHEN AND EQUIPMENT DESIGN

10.40 Some important points to be borne in mind when kitchen design is being considered:—

— the layout should allow for easy access to all areas for effective cleaning;

— adequate ventilation should be provided to prevent condensation;

— work surfaces should be impermeable and easy to clean;

— there should be clear separation of preparation areas eg between raw meat and cooked foods to avoid cross-contamination.

We recommend to the House Builders Federation, the Royal Institute of British Architects and manufacturers and fitters of domestic kitchens, that they should pay attention to the microbiological safety of the kitchens they design or install (R(II)10.12).

CLEANING

10.41 Where a kitchen is too small to provide separate areas for preparing raw meat, vegetables and cooked foods, the preparation area should be thoroughly cleaned between its use for different types of food. Studies of contamination in domestic kitchens have indicated that wet cloths, and cleaning utensils, as well as hands and implements and surfaces in contact with food may play a significant part in cross-contamination. It is important to keep food preparation surfaces dry. The following practices should be followed:—

— cloths should be kept clean and dry;

— cloths should be disinfected or boiled at frequent intervals;

— chopping boards and other surfaces should be thoroughly cleaned and treated with suitably diluted disinfectant;

— wooden chopping boards, with worn or damaged surfaces which cannot be properly cleaned, may present a particular hazard and should not be used;

— full use should be made of disposable paper towels to wipe surfaces, particularly where raw meat or poultry are involved;

— towels for hand drying should not be used for drying dishes and vice versa.

10.42 Automatic dishwashers which use very hot water, a strong detergent and air drying, are excellent for decontaminating dishes and utensils. For hand washing-up, the hottest possible water, with detergent, should be used and the water should be changed frequently. Ideally the dishes should be left to drip dry. If tea towels are used they should be clean and dry.

HOUSEHOLD PETS

10.43 Many households have domestic pets. It is a reasonable supposition that, in certain circumstances, pets can present a hazard to human health. It is therefore important that, whenever possible, pets should be excluded from areas where food is stored or prepared. When this cannot be achieved, extra care should be taken to clean and, if necessary, disinfect surfaces on which food is prepared or handled.

10.44 Some pets are fed on material such as meat and offal which is unsuitable for human consumption and presents a particular hazard of cross-contamination. Such food should be wrapped and kept separate from the household food. Dry pet food should also be stored separately. Opened tins of pet food should be used up as soon as possible.

10.45 Dishes, spoons and knives etc which are used to serve pet food should be washed and stored separately. Trays of cat litter should never be kept in the kitchen.

WASTE DISPOSAL

10.46 Waste material often includes contaminated products and provides an obvious breeding ground for bacteria. It should be placed in bags tied with a bag tie and removed from the kitchen frequently.

INFORMATION ON FOOD SAFETY

10.47 We welcome the government publication "Food Safety: A Guide from HM Government" and commend its wide circulation. However, we consider that the cartoon format of "Clean Food", produced by the Department of Health for food handlers in the catering industry, and of some local authority publications, transmits the message more simply and effectively. **We therefore recommend that consideration should be given to revising the format of future versions of "Food Safety: A Guide from HM Government"** (R(II)10.13).

10.48 The "Clean Food" booklet has been translated by a number of health authorities into other languages and we understand that the Government is similarly considering the possibility of versions of the "Food Safety: A Guide from HM Government" booklet aimed at ethnic minorities. **We welcome this and recommend that food safety information and advice should be more readily available to groups for whom English is not their first language** (R(II)10.14).

10.49 **We recommend that the consumer advice in paragraphs 10.7, 10.9, 10.18, 10.21, 10.33, 10.35, 10.37, 10.39 and 10.41 should also be incorporated in future versions of "Food Safety: A Guide from HM Government" where this is not already the case** (R(II)10.15).

ADVICE TO PARTICULARLY VULNERABLE GROUPS

10.50 We consider that there is a need for advice directed at those who may be more vulnerable to particular foodborne organisms eg pregnant women, very young children and elderly people. Such advice could be made available through government publications, and disseminated through GP waiting rooms, maternity and child welfare clinics, out-patient departments and by health visitors. **We recommend that the Government should consider arrangements for providing more readily available advice to those who are more vulnerable to particular foodborne organisms** (R(II)10.16).

ANNEX 10.1

CONSUMER ADVICE
LEAFLETS AND VIDEOS ON THE
MICROBIOLOGICAL SAFETY OF FOOD

1 LEAFLETS

1.1 "Food Safety: A Guide from HM Government" available free of charge from Food Sense, LONDON SE99 7TT.

1.2 Non-Government organisations, such as large supermarket chains, regularly produce leaflets on food safety and hygiene issues. The Food Safety Advisory Committee (sponsored by ASDA, Gateway, Morrisons, Safeway, Sainsburys and TESCO) produce leaflets as follows:—

(i) Safe Food

(ii) The Good Food Safety Guide

(iii) A Consumer's Guide to the Safe Handling of Food in Shops

(iv) Fridge and Freezer Safety Pack

2 VIDEOS

2.1 Two Government videos are available:—

— "Food Safety in the Kitchen"

— "Kate's Party"

The videos can be obtained on loan from CFL Vision, PO Box 35, Wetherby, Yorks LS23 7EX.

CHAPTER 11

EDUCATION AND TRAINING

INTRODUCTION

11.1 We stated in the introduction to Part I that the need for training and re-training of managers, food handlers, inspectors, and in fact of everyone involved in the food chain had repeatedly emerged during our investigations; that pattern has continued during our subsequent work.

11.2 We have drawn attention to particular education and training needs at various places in both parts of our report. Here we draw together the main points. In summary, it is hard to over-state the potential which appropriate education and training have to offer for the maintenance of food safety. If those involved in the food chain — which includes all of us as consumers — had a greater awareness of where the true risks lie and of the available safeguards, we are confident that the current incidence of foodborne illness would be very substantially reduced. However, the qualification should be added that one cannot rely on education and training alone to provide all that is needed. Thus what we recommend in this chapter must not be taken to detract from the need, expressed elsewhere in our report, for the effective monitoring and control of the food chain.

11.3 As we have already noted (Part II, paragraph 2.16), one of the most important elements in effective food safety is awareness of the potential risks and the precautions which can be taken. It is against that background that we recommended in Part I that DH and MAFF consider arrangements for providing simple but informative briefing to the public and the media (Part I, paragraph 3.45) and that efforts be made to provide epidemiological data from veterinary and human sources in simplified form (Part I, paragraphs 3.43 and 3.44 respectively). It is of the greatest importance that confidence can be placed in these data.

11.4 Another important element in effective food safety is sound advice on best practice. In Part II, paragraphs 10.47-10.50 we comment on the information available to the public on good hygiene practice.

FOOD HYGIENE IN THE EDUCATION SECTOR

11.5 Education is a lifelong process, starting in the home. Parents have a responsibility to ensure that their children are made aware of the need for good personal hygiene and careful handling of food from an early age.

Schools

11.6 In schools food hygiene has usually been taught as part of a home economics course. In England and Wales, all 11-14 year olds in mixed sex schools and in girls' schools have taken it but it has not routinely been taught in all boys' schools. Home economics is not included in the ten foundation subjects of the National Curriculum established under the Education Reform Act 1988. It could be included among non-foundation subjects but there will be keen competition for curriculum time. In Scotland, pupils are introduced to aspects of home economics in the later stages of primary schooling; subsequently all pupils will study home economics as part of the S1 and S2 common course (for pupils aged 12-14). In Northern Ireland, home economics is taught in the secondary sector. It is offered to all pupils in girls' schools in years one and two and frequently year three, and in the majority of mixed sex schools in the same manner. Few boys' schools offer the subject.

11.7 Science would be the best subject-area for teaching food hygiene if appropriate examples were included. The National Curriculum for Science in England and Wales is now approved. It includes an attainment target entitled "Processes of Life" under which food hygiene-related issues will be addressed. A small element of microbiology, which is expected to enable pupils to understand ways in which health may be affected by microbes, will be taught in key stage 3 (approximately 12-14 years). Details are fairly broad:

> ". . . through the use of a range of secondary sources they [the pupils] should extend the study of the human life-cycle and ways in which the healthy functioning of the body may be disrupted by diet, lifestyle, bacteria and viruses, and the use and abuse of medicines and drugs."

11.8 The Scottish Examination Board and the Northern Ireland Council for Examination and Assessment courses in Biology, Home Economics and Health Studies contain specific elements related to microbiology, food science and hygiene.

11.9 It is clear that precisely what is taught in secondary schools in the United Kingdom about food hygiene will depend on the schools themselves and on the syllabuses they draw up. This means that with the keen competition for curriculum time there is a danger that at least some, if not the majority, of schools will neglect this important subject. If the potential to raise the level of awareness of the importance of hygiene amongst the next generation of food purchasers is to be realised, efforts must be made to stimulate the interest of those who will teach it. Teacher training colleges should therefore stimulate this interest by the use, inter alia, of teaching material developed for that purpose. Other opportunities for improving awareness of food hygiene arise in courses taught in colleges of further education. Appropriate examples of teaching materials need to be developed. **We recommend to Government that specific packages for the teaching of food hygiene and food safety issues be developed for teacher training colleges and for colleges of further education** (R(II)11.1).

11.10 We are aware that a number of teaching aids are available which have been developed in consultation with the National Curriculum Council. The Institution of Environmental Health Officers has devised an education pack for secondary schools related to its basic Food Hygiene Certificate. We are also aware that two food hygiene packages (comprising stickers, posters, teaching notes and videos) have been produced by DH/MAFF for use both in primary and in secondary schools.

Higher Education

11.11 We noted in Part I, paragraphs 7.11 and 7.12 that there is a developing demand for more natural, fresher, healthier and more convenient foods, which is influencing the processes used by the manufacturing industry and thereby leading to an erosion of microbiological safety margins. We also noted the consequent need for greater care on the part of the distributor, retailer and caterer in handling such products. In this increasingly complex situation it is ever more important that the higher education system should provide enough qualified experts for the food industry and for central and local Government to meet their responsibilities. It would be unfortunate if the many initiatives now being undertaken in the cause of improved food hygiene were undermined by a lack of suitable personnel to implement them.

11.12 A number of polytechnics, universities and colleges already offer food science and technology degrees and these provide the basic and applied aspects of food microbiology needed by those involved in the food industry. **We recommend**

156

that the Government ensures sufficient capacity exists in institutes of higher education to meet the increased demand for appropriately qualified graduates in food microbiology, science and technology (R(II)11.2).

TRAINING
Food Handlers

11.13 Some food businesses, especially the larger ones, provide training for their staff. Local authorities and other bodies run a wide range of courses which offer employers a great deal of choice in deciding how their staff should be trained. Nevertheless, the lack of hygiene awareness amongst both staff and management has been shown by the Audit Commission survey (see Part II, paragraphs 1.22 and 1.23) to be one of the commonest factors leading to a high health risk.

11.14 Probably the single most important measure to flow from the Food Safety Act 1990 will be the requirement that people handling food should be trained. In Part I, paragraphs 7.27-7.29 we set out, in the context of food manufacturing, the following general points of principle on how this requirement might be implemented: "Managers and supervisors must be properly trained as they need to understand the microbiologically important aspects of the processes for which they are responsible. We therefore recommend that management should take explicit responsibility for food safety training;" and "In each company, management should designate, for each manufacturing stage where it is appropriate, identified individuals to be responsible for food safety training". We consider that these comments are equally valid for other parts of the food industry. Following further consideration, our detailed comments on this issue, as they affect the whole food chain, were conveyed to the Department of Health in response to their consultation document "Food Safety Bill: Hygiene Training for Food Handlers". A copy of our letter is annexed to this Chapter (Annex 11.1). **We recommend to Government that regulations on the training of food handlers are introduced in accordance with the framework outlined in the Committee's letter of 28 June 1990, in response to the Department of Health's consultation document (R(II)11.3).**

11.15 Specific recommendations relating to the training of managers and operators in slaughterhouses and in the transport industry are included in Part II, paragraphs 4.38, 4.44 and 10.52 respectively.

Enforcement Officers

11.16 Legislation is only effective if enforced. We have made a number of recommendations aimed at ensuring that the training of EHOs, in particular, adequately takes account of the need for:

— evenness of enforcement (Part I, paragraph 4.43(b));

— effective and coherent action to control food poisoning outbreaks (Part I, paragraph 4.28(c));

— knowledge of revised arrangements both for overseeing public health at local level and for the notification of communicable disease (Part I, paragraph 4.43(c));

— knowledge of food microbiology, food technology and food control systems, including the HACCP system sufficient to know when it is appropriate, and the need to seek expert advice (Part I, paragraph 7.31);

— knowledge of the particular requirements of small food processing enterprises (Part I, paragraph 8.11);

— knowledge of the principles involved in the operation of refrigerated vehicles (Part II, paragraph 7.32).

The above list is extensive if not positively daunting. It illustrates the wide-ranging responsibilities which EHOs have for food law enforcement; and this is, of course, only part of their duties.

11.17 In order to ease the burden on EHOs, we advocated in Part I, paragraph 9.15 the development of a new cadre of specialist food technicians to assist them. In addition, **we recommend to the Audit Commission that in their current study of the patterns and structure of food law enforcement in England and Wales, they consider the diversity of training required by EHOs** (R(II)11.4).

Consultants in Communicable Disease Control

11.18 In our consideration of the arrangements in England and Wales for the surveillance and control of foodborne illness at the local level we highlighted the pivotal role of the newly created post of Consultant in Communicable Disease Control (CCDC). We felt the recruitment and training of CCDCs should be pursued with vigour and we therefore wrote to the Secretary of State for Health outlining our views (Part I, Annex 4.2). In particular we noted that "if the CCDCs are to command the respect necessary for the effective discharge of their duties they will need training in epidemiology, microbiology and infectious disease control as well as in management". We are pleased to note that, for the 1990/91 financial year, £283,000 pump-priming finance has been made available from the Health Authority central fund for short-term training of CCDCs, and that £164,000 has been allocated to Regional Health Authorities for course fees and £119,000 to CDSC to develop a training module for these consultants. In Northern Ireland there is already a CCDC in each Health Board, but there is a need to provide opportunities for refresher training to ensure that the CCDCs are kept up to date. In Scotland there is a Consultant in Public Health Medicine with responsibility for communicable disease control — a post analogous to the CCDC — in each Health Board. Particular attention is being focused in Scotland on training in this aspect of public health, and a number of initiatives to aid training and updating are under way. **We recommend that the Government keep the appropriate teaching of CCDCs under review in order to ensure a sufficient commitment of funds to train and re-train CCDCs to enable them effectively to undertake their responsibilities** (R(II)11.5).

Schools of Public Health

11.19 Where the kind of training we are discussing in this Chapter is directed at professionals working in public health, we would expect that schools of public health would have an important role to play.

Food Examiners

11.20 The Food Safety Act 1990 for the first time recognises 'food examiners' separately from public analysts. Food examiners will be the individuals to whom an enforcement officer must submit any sample he has obtained for enforcement purposes (ie for use as evidence in any court proceedings under the Act) if he considers the sample should undergo microbiological examination. Under proposed Regulations to be made under the Act, qualifications will be prescribed for food examiners. The intention of the provisions is to ensure that the microbiological examination of food is carried out to a high standard, and to ensure that the competence of those who give a view on the result is not open to question. We support these aims.

Veterinary Surgeons

11.20 We noted at Part II, paragraph 4.17 the need for Official Veterinary Surgeons to undergo a dedicated programme of training and continuing in-job development if they are to apply the new arrangements proposed by the EC Commission. More generally we feel it important for veterinary surgeons to have a sound basic knowledge of public health issues relevant to veterinary medicine. We therefore welcome the initiative being undertaken by the Royal College of Veterinary Surgeons in establishing an undergraduate course covering this issue.

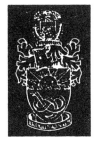

Professor Sir Mark Richmond
Sc.D., F.R.S.
Vice-Chancellor

FROM THE VICE-CHANCELLOR · THE UNIVERSITY · MANCHESTER · M13 9PL

Telephone : 061 - 275 2010

Miss K Hayes   28 June 1990
Department of Health
Room 619 Eileen House
80-94 Newington Causeway
London SE1 6EX

Dear Miss Hayes

FOOD SAFETY BILL: HYGIENE TRAINING FOR FOOD HANDLERS

I am writing to let you know the views of the Committee on Microbiological Safety of Food on the consultation document on the Government's proposal to require persons involved in food business to be trained.

Since the writing of Part I of its Report the Committee has considered the Consultation Document sent out under cover of a letter from Mr Freeman in December 1989 and has the following comments.

As indicated in Part I of our Report published on 15 February 1990, the Committee on the Microbiological Safety of Food welcomes the Government's proposals to take powers to provide for the training of those who handle food commercially, and is aware of and endorses the efforts already in hand within Government to assess existing provisions for training and to identify training needs.

We would wish to re-emphasise what we said in Part I of our Report that management is responsible for food hygiene. When improving practice by training it is important to ensure at the outset that management is committed to the programme and supportive of its aims. In this connection it is in our view essential that there is a requirement for management to keep a record of training. We also feel that programmes of training should include senior management with direct line management responsibility and that they are adequately trained before junior and more transient staff.

One practical measure which we believe would assist in putting these general principles into practice would be to require those managing food businesses to produce a written statement of their policy on food hygiene including training. This would oblige all employers and managers to think positively about their responsibilities in relation to the standards of hygiene in their businesses, and about the best way of maintaining high standards and communicating them to their staff.

In larger concerns with diverse operations statements should be provided for each area of work. Managers should satisfy themselves that their employees understand that statement before they commence work. This would help to ensure that all staff have been instructed in observing certain basic practices before being allowed to handle food. The statements should also be available for inspection by enforcement officers.

Within the framework outlined in this preamble, we have the following detailed comments on the questions raised in the consultation document.

Scope of Regulations

The Committee would wish to see the regulations covering the manufacturing, retailing and catering sections of the food industry, as well as other organizations which supply food during the course of business such as hospitals or schools. When such regulations are drawn up they should also include street traders. Nevertheless the Committee recognises that there are other areas, in particular "meals on wheels", but also "one-off" or less regular events such as charity fetes, church functions etc, where poor hygiene practices could put the public health equally at risk. In these cases, the fact that people are involved on a voluntary basis makes it much less appropriate to impose a requirement for training, even where it would be possible to do so within the scope of the enabling powers in the Bill. The danger is that such a requirement would be likely to reduce severely the number of people involved in these activities which have an important social function in the local community.

The Committee therefore recommends that where there is an umbrella organization coordinating volunteers on a regular basis eg WRVS providing volunteers to cook and distribute 'meals on wheels' on behalf of a local authority, there should be a requirement for at least one person in that organization at a local level to have undergone food hygiene training. We, however, look to the educational system backed up by information and guidance leaflets to provide the general public with the knowledge of good hygiene practice. This should commence in schools (we would like this subject as part of the core curriculum), but should be reinforced periodically by leaflets and general campaigns. Specialised leaflets covering specific situations eg large scale catering from a domestic kitchen for particular events, such as a wedding reception. The latter would be of particular benefit to those involved in catering in the voluntary sector.

With regard to possible exclusions, the Committee agrees in principle that where a food business poses only a minimal risk to health, those involved should not be required to undergo hygiene training. In practice the Committee agrees with most of the exclusions proposed by the Government, except that proposed for businesses dealing in wet fish. Those businesses selling wet fish usually also sell shell fish, and increasingly they stock other ready to eat products, a combination which the Committee considers may pose more than a minimal risk to health.

Whilst agreeing with the Government that the regulations should apply to all those who handle food directly, the Committee strongly believes that the regulations should also apply to their immediate supervisors and to their managers. There would also be benefit in extending the training requirement to maintenance and cleaning staff and others who may come into contact with production areas, particuarly those servicing machinery, so as to ensure that they behave with proper attention to food hygiene.

Management should give a lead in best practice to their junior staff. We therefore feel that programmes of training should start with senior management and should ensure that they are adequately trained before junior and more transient staff. We recognise that part-time working and temporary employment because of fluctuating business pose particular problems. The Committee does not think it would be realistic to impose formal training requirements on casual staff. Nevertheless all employees including "casuals" should receive the necessary induction training even if it is only very basic training on the "house rules" from their immediate supervisor. Clearly this places an added onus on a supervisor responsible for the work of casual staff. It is important therefore to ensure that the numbers of casual staff for whom a supervisor is expected to provide induction training and subsequent supervision is realistic. These basic rules could be included in the business' written statement of hygiene policy. Managers should satisfy themselves that employees understand the statement before they start employment.

Basic training requirement and further training

We have already drawn attention above to the importance we attach to a well trained and committed management in ensuring high hygienic standards within the food industry. Whatever training requirements are laid down in regulations we feel it is important that all organizations concerned with the validation of courses for those entering the food industry should ensure that the syllabuses, including those of courses for managers, include food hygiene.

The Committee accepts that the proposal for a basic minimum standard of training achievable in 6 hours for the majority of those involved in the food industry is all that can be reasonably achieved in legislation. However, we envisage that further training will inevitably be needed for those workers carrying out more than basic jobs. This could be provided by appropriate agencies with specialist knowledge of particular areas consulting with food businesses to meet their particular needs.

A requirement for a written statement of food hygiene policy such as we have suggested above would confer the flexibility to specify for each job within an organization the training beyond the minimum specified in regulations which was appropriate, and provide a basis for discussion between the organization and enforcement authorities about whether the employees in that organization were adequately trained.

If high standards of food hygiene are to be maintained, we also see a need for refresher and updating training as necessary, which could also be built into a written statement of hygiene policy, and for adequate supervision to ensure that knowledge is put into practice.

Methods of teaching and assessment

From a practical point of view, large numbers of training opportunities are going to be required once regulations imposing a training requirement are brought into force. We therefore welcome the Government's intention to build on what is currently available, and not to specify the method of teaching in regulations.

The NCVQ provides a framework for inclusion of a wide range of training schemes. However, it is essential that whatever training is provided for inclusion in the NCVQ framework there should be arrangements to guarantee and monitor standards. This is necessary both for employers to be sure that the training provided is adequate and for EHOs checking that training requirements are being met. We recommend that those requiring food hygiene training should enrol in courses "approved" for inclusion by NCVQ. We also recommend that there should be a register held by NCVQ of all companies and organizations carrying out training courses in food hygiene conforming with the Regulations.

Records of training

As indicated above the Committee believes it is highly desirable for management to keep a record of training. The setting up of a validation body for relevant courses as suggested would allow employers continued flexibility about how they meet the training needs of their employees and at the same time would ensure common standards for enforcement purposes. In respect of the options in paragraph 10 of the consultation document the committee favours option (iv) as a transitional arrangment leading to option (i) in the longer term.

Implementation period

The Committee is of the view that management should be obliged to comply with the new legislation in the minimum possible time and in any event we consider that this should be within 12 months of the introduction of the new legislation.

In respect of training of newly recruited staff the committee recognises that there are likely to be constraints locally regarding the availability of places on training courses. However, we think 6 weeks a reasonable period within which new staff should be trained independently of induction training provided at the start of employment.

If our suggestion that food businesses be required to produce a written statement of their food hygiene policy is taken up, managers will be required to satisfy themselves that their employees understand the statement before they commence work. This will ensure that all staff are instructed in observing certain basic principles before being allowed to handle food.

Yours sincerely

Professor Sir Mark Richmond Sc.D F.R.S.
Chairman Committee on Microbiological Safety of Food

162

CHAPTER 12

RESEARCH

INTRODUCTION

12.1 Research and surveillance provide the basis used to inform policies and decision-making by Government and industry in the area of food safety. We considered surveillance in detail in Chapter 5 of Part I and in Chapters 3 and 4 of this Part of our Report. Here we deal with research.

RESEARCH COMMISSIONING

12.2 Food safety research is sponsored in the public sector by the Agriculture and Health Departments, which commission work directly, and by the Department of Education and Science (DES), which funds the Agricultural and Food Research Council (AFRC) and the Medical Research Council (MRC). DH also funds the Public Health Laboratory Service (PHLS) which, like the AFRC and the MRC, is also able to determine programmes of work using funds received from central Government.

12.3 The expenditure on research relevant to the microbiological safety of food during 1990/91 is expected to be:

		£ million
MAFF	directly commissioned	4.6[1]
DAFS[2]	directly commissioned	0.2
DANI[3]	directly commissioned	0.7
DH	directly commissioned PHLS block funding	0.1 2.0[4]
DES	AFRC block funding MRC block funding	1 0 0.1
Total		8.7

Notes:
[1] This figure excludes research undertaken by the State Veterinary Service on zoonoses in animals
[2] Department of Agriculture & Fisheries for Scotland
[3] Department of Agriculture for Northern Ireland
[4] This figure covers research and surveillance work undertaken by the PHLS but excludes diagnostic work and work on outbreaks of foodborne illness.

12.4 In the private sector a few large companies in the food processing, distributing and catering industries have their own research departments. They and others also commission research externally, in particular from AFRC, the four food research associations, and the universities and polytechnics. Much of this research is confidential to the companies concerned, although some is published from time to time. In general the emphasis is on the development of new or improved products and processes. Companies do, however, also initiate substantial research programmes to help them meet their responsibility to produce safe and wholesome food. The private sector spending on research into the microbiological safety of food is not centrally collated and its magnitude cannot therefore readily be assessed.

COORDINATION OF RESEARCH WORK

12.5 The Agriculture Departments and the AFRC recognise the need for a coordinated approach to the allocation of funds for research and consequently have developed a comprehensive consultative machinery for deciding on the research priorities for agriculture and food. This co-ordinating function is performed by the Priorities Board for Research and Development in Agriculture and Food. It comprises mainly independent members with interests covering the whole food chain. The Board provides strategic advice to the UK Agriculture Ministers and to the Chairman of the AFRC on the balance and direction of their research programme as a whole. Under recently revised arrangements, the Board is to be supported by a number of Advisory Sectoral Groups (ASGs) which are independently chaired and made up of representatives from the main public and private bodies funding R&D in each sector. As well as advising the Priorities Board, each ASG therefore provides a means by which Government and industry can coordinate their respective research efforts. There is an ASG for Food covering all aspects of safety and nutrition, which will include members drawn from DH, industry and the relevant consumer organisations.

12.6 MAFF and DH also coordinate their work through a range of other committees. In 1987 they set up a 'Microbiological Forum' to discuss long term research needs and to ensure that the programmes which they sponsored were well coordinated. Representatives of the PHLS and the food industry as well as members of the Departments attend meetings of this group. We have been told by the Departments that they intend to link this arrangement with the new microbiological surveillance committee structure (see Part II, paragraph 1.21(b)). It is clearly important that coordination should continue and that research and surveillance should be properly integrated. **We therefore recommend that Departments should set up a research sub-group of the new Steering Group on the Microbiological Safety of Food; that it should include amongst its membership representatives of the MRC and AFRC, and that this new subgroup should be responsible for coordinating research programmes and keeping them under review (R(II)12.1).**

12.7 Through its programmes of research and surveillance the food industry as a whole clearly possesses considerable amounts of data on the microbiological safety of a wide variety of products. We believe that more of this data could be put into the public domain without harm to the commercial interests of the companies which have paid for the work. As noted in paragraph 12.5 above, the ASG for Food will bring together representatives of those funding in both the private and public sector. The ASG could, in our view, usefully be used as the forum in which data and plans are shared. Duplication of work with the proposed research sub-group would of course need to be avoided under any such arrangements. **We recommend that the Advisory Sectoral Group for Food should establish a mechanism for collating industry's research plans and results, as far as is practicable within the constraints of commercial confidentiality; and that Departments should arrange for this information and the views of the Advisory Sectoral Group to be promptly passed to the proposed research sub-group of the Steering Group on the Microbiological Safety of Food (R(II)12.2).**

RESEARCH AIMS AND PRIORITIES IDENTIFIED BY THE COMMITTEE

12.8 The Committee has identified a need for research at various points in both parts of our Report. Much of it falls under the following broad heads:—

(i) rapid, sensitive and cheap methods for detecting and identifying pathogens;

(ii) fundamental studies on the growth, survival and death of pathogens in food and the relevant environment;

(iii) fundamental studies of infective doses, infectivity and the mechanisms of microbial pathogenicity;

(iv) effective temperature history indicators to show whether food has been exposed to inappropriate storage temperatures.

12.9 In addition to these broad areas of research, we also identify a number of more specific topics we would wish to see supported:—

(i) the incidence of gastrointestinal disease in human population;

(ii) the virulence of relevant listeria species and how they infect and cause disease in humans;

(iii) the transmissibility of salmonella, particularly in eggs and poultry;

(iv) the transmissibility of verocytotoxin producing *Escherichia coli;*

(v) the depuration of small round structured viruses (SRSVs) in bivalve molluscs.

RESEARCH AIMS AND PRIORITIES IDENTIFIED BY PUBLIC BODIES

12.10 Those of the research priorities of MAFF that are relevant to the microbiological safety of food are set out in Annex 12.1 to this Chapter. This Annex is an extract from MAFF's "Food research strategy and requirements document 1991/92", issued in August 1990. We welcome the aims set out in this document. It identifies as particular priorities the potential for growth in food of newly identified pathogens, the mechanisms leading to the development of pathogenicity in food microorganisms, and the population dynamics underlying the survival of pathogens in food. The document also sets out three main initiatives as priorities for funding:

— establishing the conditions leading to growth, or inhibition of growth, of pathogens;

— developing predictive modelling of the growth of pathogens;

— developing methods for the surveillance and detection of pathogens, in particular methods for rapid detection and screening.

A major initiative on the second of these topics is already under way.

12.11 DAFS and DANI have similar research aims and priorities to those of MAFF. These are applied in the particular context of each country's social and economic needs.

12.12 Similarly, we welcome the AFRC's declared priorities for research on the microbiological safety of food. In the coming year they are likely to focus on:

— the physiology of emerging food pathogens;

— the establishment of a ribosomal ribonucleic acid (rRNA) sequence database; this will aid design of DNA probes against unique rRNA targets and will complement other work on the rapid detection and identification of foodborne pathogens;

— understanding the mechanisms underlying microbial inactivation and recovery;

— the genetic relatedness of toxigenic and non-toxigenic bacteria, especially in instances where the latter express toxins normally associated with other toxic species.

12.13 The DH directly funds some research related to the microbiological safety of food, and the PHLS uses its block funding from DH to undertake both human and food surveillance and microbiological research on food and water pathogens. It is part of the PHLS's remit to support DH's policies to improve the health and wellbeing of the population, to prevent illness and, in particular, to support the Department's policies on food safety, food hygiene, foodborne illness and microbiological contamination of food. DH has identified eight main areas where it considers that research needs to be carried out:—

— ascertainment of the true incidence of infectious gastrointestinal foodborne disease in the community (for further details see Part II, paragraph 1.21(a));

— how listeria infects the human body and the part food may play as a vehicle of infection;

— source, transmission and control of campylobacter;

— methods of determining the presence of Verocytotoxin-producing *Escherichia coli* in food;

— rapid methods for detecting pathogenic organisms;

— transmission and control of salmonella;

— identification and assessment of emerging pathogens;

— microbiological consequences of new food processes.

ASSESSMENT OF THE PLANS OF BODIES IN THE PUBLIC SECTOR

12.14 We think it important that all the bodies with a role in the funding of research on food safety should have appropriately co-ordinated strategies. This is generally the case, although it appears that the MRC is not at this time significantly involved in supporting work on food safety. However, we understand that the MRC has decided to mount a review of its research programmes on infection, particularly concentrating on bacterial infection, during the coming year with a view to determining future priorities. We welcome this and urge the MRC to take up the recommendation in paragraph 12.16 below.

12.15 We note with approval MAFF's decision to publish a list of its research priorities (see paragraph 12.10 above). We believe it is important that research strategies should be published in this way. **We recommend that all those funding public sector research on the microbiological safety of food should develop appropriate research strategies and indicate how they are to be implemented** (R(II)12.3).

12.16 The research priorities identified by the Committee (see paragraphs 12.8 and 12.9) are, with a few exceptions, covered by one or other of the public bodies in their future research programmes. Indeed the work which DH has now instigated on the ascertainment of the true incidence of infectious gastrointestinal foodborne disease in the community is a direct response to the recommendation we made at Part I, paragraphs 3.35 and 3.36. Where it is not apparent that the priorities we have identified are being covered in Departments' plans, as is the case with the depuration of SRSVs in bivalve molluscs and with temperature history indicators, we have made recommendations to this effect in our consideration of the parts of the food chain where the problems arise (see Part II, paragraphs 6.13 and 10.20 respectively). The one priority area which is not the subject of a specific recommendation elsewhere relates to various aspects of the pathogenicity of microorganisms. **We therefore recommend that the MRC take forward work on fundamental studies of infective doses, infectivity and mechanisms of microbial pathogenicity as soon as possible** (R(II)12.4).

COLLABORATION BETWEEN THE PUBLIC AND PRIVATE SECTORS

12.17 We understand that collaborative research involving both the public and the private sectors is already being carried out under the 'LINK' programme, though few projects supported to date specifically cover the microbiological safety of food. In addition individual laboratories and institutes are collaborating with their leading counterparts overseas. We believe that this can only lead to greater value for money and a more rapid advancement of the science base than would otherwise be possible. **We recommend that every opportunity be taken to develop both national and international collaborative research programmes on the microbiological safety of food** (R(II)12.5).

ANNEX 12.1

EXTRACTS FROM "FOOD RESEARCH STRATEGY AND REQUIREMENTS DOCUMENT 1991/92" OF THE MINISTRY OF AGRICULTURE, FISHERIES AND FOOD

Food Safety and Applied Nutrition

2.1 The research commissioned by MAFF provides the major input into the scientific basis for consumer protection, the elaboration of a national food policy, and its effective implementation through statutory or non-statutory controls.

The Ministry through its Food Safety Directorate has the responsibility to protect the public by promoting food safety. It also has the responsibility to protect the public from being defrauded. This consumer protection activity requires scientific information relating to food composition, adulteration and authenticity.

The specific aims are:

i. to safeguard food safety with respect to pathogenic microorganisms in food;

ii. to safeguard food safety with respect to adventitious chemicals and their residues in food;

iii. to assess the nutrient content of the food supply, consumer intakes of nutrients, and the significance of these intakes;

iv. to safeguard the authenticity of foods and prevent adulteration;

v. to provide scientific and technical advice to expert Committees in MAFF and other Departments and to Ministers on the use of chemicals in food and on the presence of chemicals in food arising from adventitious or accidental causes;

vi. to advise on the likely exposure of the UK population, including critical groups, to food chemicals and to propose how risk management for food chemicals can best be carried out;

vii. to maintain a body of scientific expertise and back-up information to respond to the needs in this area and in particular to enable appropriate responses to be made to new identified hazards in the food chain, including those arising from emergencies.

PATHOGENIC MICROORGANISMS

Introduction

4.1 The Ministry's policy is to ensure that food as consumed contains insufficient numbers of pathogenic microorganisms to cause foodborne infections. In addition, the numbers of pathogenic microorganisms in or on raw materials should be as low as practicable. However, laying down microbiological standards in terms of limits on numbers of particular microorganisms is not regarded as the best approach for control purposes. The objective is to identify for each type of food the hygiene controls most appropriate according to a Hazard Analysis and Critical Control Point (HACCP) system. Such knowledge is also required in order to lay down control measures in UK regulations, in Codes of Practice, to negotiate appropriate measures in EC Directives and Regulations, and appropriate Codex Alimentarius hygiene standards.

Conditions Leading to Growth or Inhibition of Growth of Pathogens

4.2 In order to meet these needs research is necessary into the following topics:—

— the effect of processing conditions such as heat, cold, water activity, pH, atmosphere, packaging on the growth or inhibition of growth on food pathogenic microorganisms;

— the effectiveness of various processes on controlling microbial growth, eg microwave and ohmic heating, irradiation, aseptic processing, sous-vide, cook-chill etc;

— modelling of heat or cold penetration or generation in complex food substrates.

Predictive Modelling

4.3 A major initiative funded by MAFF which is presently underway, and which will continue until 1993, is designed to provide a unique data base and expert system to predict the growth and inhibition of growth of the principal pathogenic microorganisms in foods and model systems. This overall initiative is directed by a Programme Manager, appointed by MAFF, and is supervised by an overall Programme Management Committee. The present work programme of this initiative, and the principal contractors, are shown in Appendix 1 (not attached as part of this Report).

The overall aim is to develop accurate mathematical models which will enable legislators and the food industry to assess the risk of growth of specific micro-organisms in new food formulations and processes. Specific further research requirements for this initiative are identified by the Programme Manager. Any further requirements are likely to fall into the areas of:

— more accurate models, particularly those which are better able to predict the recovery of sub-lethally injured organisms;

— more efficient means of generating the data for evaluating the accuracy of the models used.

Contractors who feel they have the potential for contributing successfully to this initiative should contact the Programme Manager through the Chief Scientists' Group.

Surveillance and Detection of Pathogens

4.4 Microbiological surveillance of food is essential to measure the effectiveness of food hygiene controls. Such surveillance can provide causal links between actual food poisoning outbreaks as well as discounting purported links. Surveillance will also confirm the success of existing hygiene controls and identify the need for improvements. Consequently there is a continuing need for the development of improved and more rapid methods of analysis for microorganisms in food.

Specific requirements are:
— rapid methods which will eliminate the need for pre-extraction and enrichment of microorganisms from food;

— improved methods for the isolation and concentration of microorganisms from food;

— methods suitable for the rapid detection and screening of pathogenic microorganisms (specific identification is not necessarily required);

— methods suitable for the specific detection of pathogenic strains of selected food organisms (the priority is not necessarily for very rapid methods, specificity is a more important criterion);

— methods suitable for on-line detection.

Microorganisms of particular interest include pathogenic strains of Salmonella, Campylobacter and Listeria together with so-called "emerging" pathogens such as Yersinia and E.coli 0157. The potential for growth in food of other newly identified pathogens will be of particular priority for research support.

In evaluating research proposals in this field, MAFF will pay particular attention to the potential for exploitation by industry. Sole support for research in the public sector will depend on the extent to which the research objectives are dependant on private sector investment for the effective exploitation of the technologies proposed.

At a more fundamental level MAFF has an interest in understanding the mechanisms leading to the development of pathogenicity in food microorganisms, and on the population dynamics underlying survival of food pathogens. Whilst the primary responsibility for this basic research lies with the research councils, MAFF will consider supporting more applied projects in this area.

CHAPTER 13

RECOMMENDATIONS

EPIDEMIOLOGICAL SURVEILLANCE

R(II)1.1 We therefore *recommend* that the topic of eggs should be considered by the Steering Group and Advisory Committee on the Microbiological Safety of Food as soon as possible in their programmes of work. (1.13)

R(II)1.2 We reiterate most strongly our recommendation (Part I paragraph 3.46) that the PHLS should take steps to eliminate the confusion that can potentially arise from the lack of comparability between these two data series. (1.18)

R(II)1.3 We *recommend* that the Steering Group on the Microbiological Safety of Food should consult all the countries of the UK with a view to putting data collection and reporting on a commonly agreed basis. (1.19)

REGISTRATION

R(II)1.4 We therefore *recommend* that enforcement officers should take full advantage of registration in order to identify the businesses most in need of attention, and to provide them with information and advice. (1.30)

SCOTLAND

R(II)3.1 We further *recommend* that Government should work towards a common definition of food poisoning for all countries of the United Kingdom, and ideally for the whole of the European Community. (3.14)

R(II)3.2 We therefore *recommend* to the Scottish Office, that the current arrangements for national surveillance coordinators should be placed on a more formal basis, with any necessary expenses being met and an obligation to report to the Director of CD(S)U at least annually. (3.19)

R(II)3.3 We *recommend* to the Scottish Home and Health Department that the proposed linking together of general practices through the development of an existing electronic network should proceed and that infectious gastrointestinal disease be included in the diseases reported. (3.20)

R(II)3.4 We *recommend* that the Steering Group on the Microbiological Safety of Food should consider including general practices from other countries of the United Kingdom in any subsequent plans for a nationwide survey of infectious gastrointestinal disease. (3.21)

R(II)3.5 The Committee therefore *recommends* that the Scottish Home and Health Department should identify and fund a core group of laboratories explicitly to undertake public health microbiological work. (3.39)

R(II)3.6 We *recommend* that the Steering Group on the Microbiological Safety of Food should liaise with the Scottish Food Coordinating Committee on the surveillance of the microbiological safety of food in Scotland. (3.41)

R(II)3.7 We *recommend* that the Government keep the arrangements for veterinary microbiology related to food safety in Scotland under review. (3.44)

R(II)3.8 We *recommend* that the State Veterinary Service maintains arrangements which properly recognise the importance of continuing liaison with the Communicable Diseases (Scotland) Unit. (3.47)

R(II)3.9 The Committee *recommends* that the Scottish Office should set up a formal central group to ensure close liaison between health, animal health and food interests and to co-ordinate arrangements for the oversight and management of microbiological food safety matters. (3.50)

R(II)3.10 The Committee also *recommends* that the central group proposed in R(II)3.9 should be closely linked with the newly established UK Steering Group on the Microbiological Safety of Food (see Chapter 1, paragraph 1.13) which has representation from Scotland. (3.51)

R(II)3.11 We *recommend* that all the relevant UK Departments consider the need for simple and informative briefings to the public and media at appropriate intervals and should ensure that the information issued to the public and the media is consistent. (3.52)

NORTHERN IRELAND

R(II)3.12 We *recommend* to DHSS(NI) that the relevant allocation for the microbiological examination of foods by the Belfast City Hospital is clearly identified in the overall budget provided to the Eastern Health Board. (3.62)

R(II)3.13 We *recommend* that the Government should work towards a common definition of food poisoning for the whole of the UK. (3.65)

R(II)3.14 We *recommend* that consideration be given by DHSS(NI), in consultation with the Royal College of General Practitioners, to including some practices in Northern Ireland in the general practice spotter schemes existing or being developed in Great Britain. (3.69)

R(II)3.15 We *recommend* that, wherever feasible, all outbreaks in the province are reported to DHSS(NI) and summaries and statistics published at least annually that are comparable with other foodborne outbreak data in the United Kingdom. (3.70)

R(II)3.16 We *recommend* that DHSS(NI) arrange for the central collation and analysis of the results of tests on food samples taken by environmental health officers in Northern Ireland. (3.83)

R(II)3.17 We *recommend* that DHSS(NI) should collate the results of tests and surveys of food carried out by the Department of Agriculture for Northern Ireland together with those from the sampling programme undertaken by environmental health officers. (3.84)

RED MEAT

R(II)4.1 We *recommend*, once the new EC arrangements for meat inspection are agreed and ready for implementation:—

i. that the Government should ensure that provision is made

— for the training of a sufficient number of meat inspectors, Environmental Health Officers and veterinarians; and

— for the setting up of arrangements under which the disciplines involved act as a team led by the veterinary surgeon authorised for the purpose;

ii. that the appointment of the veterinary surgeon within the system should be on a longer-term and a more permanent basis; and

iii. that the State Veterinary Service should be given explicit responsibility for overseeing the meat inspection and hygiene arrangements. (4.18)

R(II)4.2 We *recommend* that abattoir managers should pay farmers a premium to take account of the cleanliness of the animals as one of the components of quality. (4.19)

R(II)4.3 We *recommend* that those carrying out antemortem inspection should devote particular attention to cull animals. (4.24)

R(II)4.4 We *recommend* that the Government should encourage technical developments in electronic tagging, and should be alert to any opportunity to put the practice to use in the control of animal disease. (4.25)

R(II)4.5 We *recommend* that all new markets and abattoirs should have wash bay facilities for lorries on site or immediately adjacent. (4.28)

R(II)4.6 We firmly *recommend* that all calves should be slaughtered on the day of arrival at the slaughterhouse. (4.31)

R(II)4.7 We *recommend* that a freshly sanitised knife be used for bleeding each animal. (4.32)

R(II)4.8 We *recommend* that the Government consider whether the practice of pithing should cease, as it introduces an unnecessary risk of contamination even if a sterilised pithing rod is used. (4.32)

R(II)4.9 We *recommend* the use of the new "inverted dressing" system for sheep which provides a much cleaner method of removing the fleece. (4.33)

R(II)4.10 Therefore, we *recommend* to slaughterhouse managers that care must be taken to wait at least six minutes after bleeding before passing the pigs into the scald tank, that the temperature of the water should be monitored closely, and that the water should be frequently changed. (4.34)

R(II)4.11 We *recommend* that attention be paid to the hygienic aspects of the design of the machinery used for washing or scrubbing pig carcases. (4.34)

R(II)4.12 We *recommend* that industry adopt the practice of tying and bagging, particularly for cattle and pigs, as soon as possible. (4.35)

R(II)4.13 We *recommend* that the oesophagus is sealed at the entrance to the rumen, which in cattle requires a rodding technique to be used. We also *recommend* that new plant should be designed to permit the use of the techniques necessary to achieve this. (4.36)

R(II)4.14 We *recommend* that in future those designating slaughter equipment should make ease of cleaning a high priority, and that management should make sure that staff are trained in the cleansing and disinfection procedures. (4.38)

R(II)4.15 We *recommend* that particular attention be given to ensuring sufficient airflow and minimum contact between carcases in chill rooms. (4.43)

R(II)4.16 We *recommend* that the industry ensures that all managers and operatives are aware of the importance of minimising contamination and the steps that should be taken to achieve this. We also *recommend* that enforcement officers should pay close attention to the hygiene implications of line speed when performing their duties and should not hesitate to insist on operations being suspended if practices are not satisfactory. (4.44)

R(II)4.17 We *recommend* the Steering Group on the Microbiological Safety of Food to consider how arrangements can best be made for the work formerly done by the Agricultural and Food Research Council on microbiological monitoring to be taken forward. (4.45)

**MILK AND
MILK PRODUCTS**

R(II)5.1 We *recommend* that the Government's new measures relating to the testing and labelling of untreated milk should be very rigorously enforced and the incidence of foodborne illness associated with the consumption of untreated milk kept closely under review. (5.28)

R(II)5.2 We *recommend* to the Government that milk and milk products originating from sheep and goats should be subjected as soon as possible to controls similar to those which apply to cows' milk and products made from it. (5.29)

R(II)5.3 We *recommend* that designers of equipment for heat treatment and bottling — including pipelines — should take proper account of the needs of hygiene, and especially of the need to enable in-place cleaning to be undertaken if at all possible. (5.36)

R(II)5.4 We *recommend* to producers the detailed advice on production of soft cheese which is set out in "Guidelines for good hygienic practice in the manufacture of soft and fresh cheeses", which was produced by the Creamery Proprietors' Association in 1988. (5.39)

R(II)5.5 We *recommend* the Government to work for the adoption of a well-founded and practical standard for the presence of L.monocytogenes in cheese which can be worked to and enforced internationally. (5.48)

R(II)5.6 We *recommend* that Government should ensure at both the national and European levels that cheese producers are made fully aware of the microbiological hazards of making cheese from untreated milk; that strict hygienic controls are laid down for the production of cheese, including monitoring the microbiological standard of the milk used; and that every step be taken through the application of the HACCP approach and end product monitoring to ensure that the cheese is microbiologically safe and is not contaminated after processing. (5.51)

R(II)5.7 We *recommend* that ways of improving the design of driers and ancilliary equipment used in the manufacture of milk powder be investigated. (5.54)

R(II)5.8 We *recommend* that manufacturers should ensure that the production of novel and composite milk products is always subject to expert assessment and close monitoring. (5.62)

FISH AND SHELLFISH

R(II)6.1 We *recommend* that the Government fund research into detection methods for small numbers of SRSVs and for hepatitis 'A' virus in molluscs. We further *recommend* that this research be followed up to evaluate and, if necessary, to improve the depuration process or to develop new techniques for the elimination of viruses from live bivalve molluscs. (6.13)

R(II)6.2 We *recommend* to the Government that research is undertaken to establish better indicators of viral contamination of water than E.coli and the other bacterial organisms currently used. (6.15)

R(II)6.3 We *recommend* to the Steering Group on the Microbiological Safety of Food that the effectiveness of the proposed EC Regulation COM(89)648 in reducing mollusc contamination and human illness should be monitored in the UK once it has been adopted and that, if the evidence warrants it, the UK Government should press for the requirements of the Regulation to be reviewed. (6.16)

R(II)6.4 We *recommend* that all processors of bivalve molluscs adopt methods that provide an effective heat process and avoid subsequent cross-contamination. (6.17)

R(II)6.5 We *recommend* that Port Health Authorities should continue their testing of imports of frozen cooked (warm water) prawns. We also *recommend* that importers be reminded that hygiene standards in the processing plants in the countries of origin are an essential ingredient in effective quality control. (6.20)

R(II)6.6 We *recommend* that, when establishing or replacing their facilities, fish farmers should install concrete raceways for the cultivation of trout, instead of mud-bottomed ponds. (6.22)

R(II)6.7 We *recommend* that, to prevent the growth of Clostridium botulinum, all producers of smoked fish ensure that salt levels are maintained at adequate levels. (6.24)

R(II)6.8 We *recommend* that the Government should update their guidelines on the handling of trout and extend them to other fish species. (6.26)

R(II)6.9 We *recommend* that persons should not be allowed to engage in the supplying of smoked fish by mail order unless they are able to demonstrate that their products will not support the growth of pathogenic microorganisms at ambient temperatures. (6.27)

R(II)6.10 We *recommend* that the Regulations which the Government has announced its intention of making on the production, storage and distribution of vacuum packed and other hermetically-sealed products should contain requirements aimed at ensuring the microbiological safety of pre-packed fish, as we understand the Government intends that they should. (6.28)

TRANSPORT

R(II)7.1 We *recommend* that the Government, in collaboration with the relevant industry and professional bodies, should produce a Code of Practice based on existing guidelines, for all transport of refrigerated foodstuffs. (7.16)

R(II)7.2 We *recommend* that the temperature requirements of the Food Hygiene (Amendment) Regulations 1990 should apply without derogation to all forms of refrigerated and insulated transport, that the Steering Group on the Microbiological Safety of Food should monitor the situation, and that the Government should consider the Food Hygiene (Amendment)Regulations 1990 to be of an interim nature and keep its requirements under careful review. (7.19)

R(II)7.3 We *recommend* to cold store operators that when new storage and loading facilities are being designed particular attention should be paid to the principles of loading pre-chilled produce into pre-cooled vehicles and adequately protecting the store/vehicle interface from higher ambient temperature. (7.22)

R(II)7.4 We *recommend* to fleet operators that temperature monitoring facilities be fitted to existing vehicles wherever possible and that such facilities should be incorporated in all new refrigerated vehicles. (7.24)

R(II)7.5 We *recommend* that Government consider the modification of domestic legislation so that the conditions set out in the ATP can be applied to domestic transport as soon as possible. (7.27)

R(II)7.6 We *recommend* that those involved in the design and construction of longer refrigerated vehicles pay particular attention to ensuring adequate temperature control. (7.29)

R(II)7.7 We *recommend* that all staff handling food during predistribution storage, loading and unloading of vehicles, and drivers of refrigerated vehicles, should receive adequate training in the principles of basic food hygiene, temperature control and product protection. (7.30)

R(II)7.8 We *recommend* to Government that knowledge on the carriage and handling of perishable foodstuffs and a basic knowledge of food hygiene be included in the tests for the Certificate of Professional Competence. (7.31)

R(II)7.9 We also *recommend* that the principles involved in the operation of refrigerated vehicles should be included in the training of environmental health officers who are responsible for enforcing legislation covering the hygiene conditions of the distribution of foods. (7.32)

RETAILING AND WHOLESALING

R(II)8.1 We *recommend* that the Government should institute discussion with wholesalers and retailers with a view to recording identifying marks for all consignments, so far as is acceptable under EC rules, at all stages as they move through the distribution chain. (8.10)

R(II)8.2 We *recommend* that the Federation of Wholesale Distributors continues to use its membership to disseminate and to promote high standards of food safety among wholesalers. (8.16)

R(II)8.3 We *recommend* to Government that further information about small wholesalers and cash-and-carry operators be obtained with a view to assessing whether specific guidance needs to be drawn up for this sector. (8.18)

R(II)8.4 We *recommend* that food manufacturers should consider including information on the handling and storage of a product on the outside of its packaging. (8.24)

R(II)8.5 We *recommend* that the Government should take the lead in consulting all interested parties and in compiling, for distribution to smaller food retailing businesses, an information pack on appropriate storage of goods and stock control. (8.25)

R(II)8.6 We *recommend* that retailers purchasing second-hand refrigeration equipment, should ensure that it is capable of achieving and maintaining the required temperatures. (8.30)

R(II)8.7 The Committee *recommend*s that there should be uniform and effective enforcement of the Food Hygiene (Amendment) Regulations 1990, so that temperature control requirements are fully met. (8.31)

R(II)8.8 We *recommend* that the relevant trade assocations should take the initiative in producing detailed guidelines on the design of premises for retail businesses. (8.35)

R(II)8.9 We *recommend* that attention should be drawn to the guidelines referred to in R(II)8.8, in the codes of practice to be issued under Section 40 of the Food Safety Act. (8.36)

R(II)8.10 We *recommend* to the Government that general requirements relating to the layout of premises retailing food be included in a future revision of the Food Hygiene (General) Regulations. (8.37)

R(II)8.11 We *recommend* the Government to bring together appropriate groups, including the Retail Consortium, to promote discussion between equipment manufacturers and retailers aimed at improving the hygienic design of equipment. (8.38)

R(II)8.12 We *recommend* to enforcement authorities that registration should be used to provide the retail sector with guidance on the Food Safety Act 1990 and the Food Hygiene Regulations, with information on training requirements and available courses, and with any future relevant guidance and information on statutory requirements and good practices. (8.41)

R(II)8.13 We *recommend* that food equipment manufacturers should look into the possibility of developing more hygienic meat slicers for use by the food industry, and that this aspect should form part of the Government-led discussions referred to in R(II)9.8. (8.45)

R(II)8.14 We reiterate the need for the licensing of those premises carrying out butchery and the processing of meat. In the meantime, in the abscence of licensing, although all food premises generally will be registered under the Food Safety Act 1990, we *recommend* that the enforcement authorities pay particular attention to those retail businesses cooking meat on their premises. (8.49)

R(II)8.15 We *recommend* to the trade associations, including the Federation of Bakers and the National Association of Master Bakers, Confectioners and Caterers, that they bring to the attention of their members the need for particularly strict hygienic practices when handling products containing meat or cream. (8.51)

R(II)8.16 The Committee *recommend*s to the Steering Group on the Microbiological Safety of Food that research should be undertaken into the contamination of unpacked foods retailed as self-service items. (8.53)

R(II)8.17 We *recommend* that, when selling ice cream which is not prepacked, retailers follow closely the guidelines produced by the Ice Cream Federation and Ice Cream Alliance. (8.60)

R(II)8.18 The Committee *recommend*s MAFF and DH to draw up guidelines for those operating farm shops; these could be disseminated by the National Farmers Union and by the enforcement authorities as part of the registration process for food premises. (8.61)

R(II)8.19 We *recommend* that enforcement authorities should pay particular attention to sales from stalls and vehicles and should ensure close liaison with other relevant enforcement authorities, so that storage and transport provisions for relevant foods supplied to such businesses are also thoroughly checked. (8.65)

R(II)8.20 We *recommend* that Government consider with industry the preparation of guidance on how to minimise risk from doorstep deliveries of food and drink, and that this guidance should be included in future versions of their food safety booklet. (8.67)

R(II)9.1 We *recommend* that caterers should follow a disciplined and carefully structured approach to the identification of hazards and control points; and that advice to caterers, which we propose in R(II)19.14 should be issued through enforcement authorities, should emphasise the importance of this approach for the safe management of catering operations. (9.10)

R(II)9.2 We *recommend* that, when EHOs inspect premises used for the sale and distribution of food to caterers, they should pay particular attention to the hygienic quality of the products and their storage and transport. (9.17)

R(II)9.3 We *recommend* that the guidelines for the catering industry referred to in R(II)9.14 should include more detailed advice on storage. (9.21)

R(II)9.4 We *recommend* that the guidelines referred to in R(II)9.14 should contain advice on the times and temperatures needed for effective cooking of different types of food. (9.24)

R(II)9.5 We *recommend* that the guidelines referred to in R(II)9.14 should include advice on the maintenance of all equipment and the methods for monitoring the temperature of refrigeration equipment. (9.27)

R(II)9.6 We *recommend* that caterers, when planning a kitchen, should consider the need to provide separate areas for clean and dirty processes, and have regard to good production flow, to reduce the risks from cross-contamination. (9.28)

R(II)9.7 We *recommend* that the guidelines referred to in R(II)9.14 should include advice on the design of kitchens which would be appropriate for catering businesses especially the small independent caterers; and that these guidelines should be used by environmental health departments in offering advice and guidance to such businesses. (9.32)

R(II)9.8 We *recommend* that the Government brings together appropriate Groups to promote discussion between UK producers and the users of catering equipment, aimed at improving the hygienic design of equipment and, in particular, at ensuring that appropriate EC design standards are agreed upon. (9.37)

R(II)9.9 We therefore *recommend* that anyone intending to open a catering business should contact their local environmental health department as early as possible, and certainly before expensive decisions on layout are taken, so that appropriate information and guidance can be provided. (9.38)

R(II)9.10 We *recommend* that environmental health departments of local authorities should be informed and involved whenever planning permission is sought for catering premises or applications made for change of use. (9.39)

R(II)9.11 We *recommend* that, for the time being, the catering industry and local authorities should use the manual "Hygiene" as a basis to improve standards throughout the industry. (9.47)

R(II)9.12 We *recommend* that the Government should incorporate advice on the use of formal notices in the codes of practice for enforcement authorities. (9.54)

R(II)9.13 We *recommend* that all enforcement authorities should institute risk assessment as a basis for proper monitoring and enforcement. We further *recommend* to the Government that guidelines on risk assessment be drawn up and issued to enforcement authorities. (9.56)

R(II)9.14 We *recommend* that the Government should take the lead in drawing up guidelines for the catering industry which include:—

a. identification of hazard points and control

b. good storage practices

c. temperatures for the effective cooking of food

d. maintenance of equipment and methods of monitoring the temperature of refrigeration equipment

e. design and planning of kitchens including provision of separate areas for clean and dirty processes

as discussed elsewhere in this Chapter, and that the enforcement authorities should then consider how to ensure that these guidelines reach individual caterers. (9.58)

R(II)9.15 The Committee *recommend*s that the Government should move to the licensing of all catering establishments, as soon as possible. (9.59)

R(II)9.16 We *recommend* that both the Steering Group and the Advisory Committee on the Microbiological Safety of Food should consider further studies on catering. (9.60)

THE CONSUMER AND THE HOME

R(II)10.1 We *recommend* that the Steering Group on the Microbiological Safety of Food should review the available information on the microbiology of the kitchen, and assess the need for further studies of the causes of contamination. (10.4)

R(II)10.2 We therefore *recommend* that chilled foods should be transported home quickly, and that much wider use should be made of cool bags/boxes. (10.10)

R(II)10.3 We *recommend* that, if their refrigerators do not have a built-in thermometer, consumers should buy a reliable thermometer and use it to monitor the temperature of the refrigerator. (10.16)

R(II)10.4 We *recommend* that the design of domestic refrigerators should include such food safety features as more precise temperature control, separated internal compartments (including a zone at 3°C), and built-in thermometers with external displays. (10.17)

R(II)10.5 We *recommend* that the Government should, in collaboration with industry, sponsor research into the development of a simple, inexpensive and reliable temperature history indicator. (10.20)

R(II)10.6 We therefore *recommend* that all manufacturers of microwave ovens should adopt a standard based on the IEC standard 705, for assessing the power rating of ovens marketed in the UK. (10.25)

R(II)10.7 We therefore *recommend* that all manufacturers of microwave ovens should label the front of the oven conspicuously with an indication of its power rating assessed in accordance with the IEC standard 705. We further *recommend* that manufacturers should display simple operating instructions conspicuously on the front of microwave ovens, on the lines of many other types of domestic appliances. (10.26)

R(II)10.8 We *recommend* that microwave oven manufacturers should inform owners of models produced before the IEC standard is adopted, of their oven's rating according to that standard. (10.29)

R(II)10.9 We *recommend* that microwave oven manufacturers should carry out more research to evaluate properly which design features most affect unevenness of heating, and should pay attention to the need for evenness of heating when designing new models. (10.30)

R(II)10.10 We *recommend* that a code of practice should be developed jointly by food manufacturers and microwave oven manufacturers, to determine a basis for establishing microwave heating instructions. (10.33)

R(II)10.11 We *recommend* that the manufacturers of microwave ovens should ensure that clear guidance on those foods which are suitable for microwave cooking, and those which are not, is included in the recipe books they usually supply with their equipment. (10.34)

R(II)10.12 We *recommend* to the House Builders Federation, the Royal Institute of British Architects and manufacturers and fitters of domestic kitchens, that they should pay attention to the microbiological safety of the kitchens they design or install. (10.40)

R(II)10.13 We therefore *recommend* that consideration should be given to revising the format of future versions of "Food Safety: A Guide from HM Government". (10.47)

R(II)10.14 We *recommend* that food safety information and advice should be more readily available to groups for whom English is not their first language. (10.48)

R(II)10.15 We *recommend* that the consumer advice in paragraphs 10.7, 10.9, 10.18, 10.21, 10.33, 10.35, 10.37, 10.39 and 10.41 should be incorporated in future versions of "Food Safety: A Guide from HM Government" where this is not already the case. (10.49)

R(II)10.16 We *recommend* that the Government should consider arrangements for providing more readily available advice to those who are more vulnerable to particular foodborne organisms. (10.50)

EDUCATION AND TRAINING

R(II)11.1 We *recommend* to Government that specific issues packages for teaching of food hygiene and food safety issues be developed for teacher training colleges and for colleges of further education. (11.9)

R(II)11.2 We *recommend* that the Government ensure sufficient capacity exists in institutes of higher education to meet the increased demand for appropriately qualified graduates in food microbiology, science and technology.(11.12)

R(II)11.3 We *recommend* to Government that Regulations on the training of food handlers are introduced in accordance with the framework outlined in the Committee's letter of 28 June 1990, in response to the Department of Health's consultation document. (11.14)

R(II)11.4 We *recommend* to the Audit Commission that in their current study of the patterns and structure of food law enforcement in England and Wales, they consider the diversity of training required by EHOs. (11.17)

R(II)11.5 We *recommend* that the Government keep the appropriate training of

CCDCs under review in order to ensure a sufficient commitment of funds to train and re-train CCDCs to enable them effectively to undertake their responsibilities. (11.18)

RESEARCH

R(II)12.1 We therefore *recommend* that Departments should set up a research sub-group of the new Steering Group on the Microbiological Safety of Food; that it should include amongst its membership representatives of the MRC and AFRC and that this new sub-group should be responsible for co-ordinating research programmes and keeping them under review. (12.6)

R(II)12.2 We *recommend* that the Advisory Sectoral Group for Food should establish a mechanism for collating industry's research plans and results, as far as is practicable within the contraints of commercial confidentiality; and that Departments should arrange for this information and the views of the Advisory Sectoral Group to be promptly passed to the proposed research sub-group of the Steering Group on the Microbiological Safety of Food. (12.7)

R(II)12.3 We *recommend* that all those funding public sector research on the microbiological safety of food should develope appropriate research strategies and indicate how they are to be implemented. (12.15)

R(II)12.4 We therefore *recommend* that the MRC take forward work on fundamental studies of infective doses, infectivity and mechanisms of microbial pathogenicity as soon as possible. (12.16)

R(II)12.5 We *recommend* that every opportunity be taken to develop both national and international collaborative research programmes on the microbiological safety of food. (12.17)

APPENDIX 1

REPORT OF THE COMMITTEE ON THE MICROBIOLOGICAL SAFETY OF FOOD
PART 1
RECOMMENDATIONS AND GOVERNMENT'S RESPONSE

FOOD BORNE ILLNESS AND EPIDEMIOLOGICAL SURVEILLANCE

RECOMMENDATION

(the numbers refer to the numbering of the recommendations and paragraphs in the Report).

R.2.1 There is an urgent need for us to understand better how listeria monocytogenes infects the human body, and what part food may play as a vehicle for infection. There is also a need to know more about the factors controlling the growth of the bacterium in different types of food so that protective measures can be taken. We *recommend* that the Government puts in hand research to answer these questions as soon as possible. (2.14)

R.3.1 We *recommend* a study of the incidence of infectious intestinal disease based on general practitioner (GP) consultations in which microbiological confirmation of the clinical diagnosis is carried out. We *recommend* that this study be set up by the Department of Health (DH) as an urgent priority. (3.35)

R.3.2 In addition we believe that the true incidence of infectious gastro-intestinal disease in the community needs to be ascertained. Thus we also *recommend* that a study including microbiological screening should be set up to provide information on the incidence of gastro-intestinal illness in the community that can be linked to a microbiological cause. This should take place, if possible, in the same areas as the GP based study. (3.36)

R.3.3 We welcome the present liaison between Communicable Disease Surveillance Centre (CDSC) and State Veterinary Service (SVS) but believe that there is a need for these links to be strengthened so that there is closer co-ordination between the CDSC and its human database and the SVS and its animal databases. This should enable the possible links between pathogens causing human disease and the same organism in food animals to be more readily established. We *recommend* that this situation [existing links between the veterinary and human systems] should be strengthened by giving PHLS a formal responsibility to collate information from human and veterinary sources to give as complete a view as possible of the current state of the microbiological contamination of humans and food animals and of any developing trends. This collation will also need to take account of the results of the food surveillance system we propose in Chapter 5. (3.39-3.41)

R.3.4 We also *recommend* that PHLS should strengthen the links between CDSC and the SVS by giving a member of CDSC staff special responsibility for zoonoses. (3.42)

RESPONSE

R.2.1 The Government has put in hand research into the incidence of listeriosis in pregnant women and is considering other research. The Public Health Laboratory Service has carried out a number of surveys of the extent of contamination of some foods with listeria monocytogenes and has recently established a network of 15 food laboratories to take the work forward in a more co-ordinated fashion.

R.3.1 and R.3.2 The Government accepts there is a need to find out more about the incidence of foodborne illness in the UK, and is considering with relevant experts how best to take this forward.

R.3.3 The Government agrees that the links between CDSC and SVS should be strengthened and that this should include moves towards co-ordination of human and veterinary databases. Some aspects of collating such information are already undertaken by the PHLS and the SVS on an informal basis.

R.3.4 This recommendation is accepted. Links already exist between PHLS and SVS which has responsibility for zoonoses.

R.3.5 A veterinary publication to complement that from the CDSC is overdue, and we *recommend* that serious consideration be given to producing a more frequent publication, analogous to the Communicable Disease Report (CDR), not less frequently than monthly. (3.43)

R.3.5 The Government accepts the need for a more frequent publication of veterinary information and will consider ways in which this might be achieved.

R.3.6 We *endorse* the decision of PHLS to reconsider the status of the CDR which at present has only a limited circulation and we welcome plans for its change to a formal publication by the end of 1990. (3.44)

R.3.6 The Government agrees on the need to publish clear information, welcomes the Committee's support and is already considering how the information can be enhanced.

With the wide interest from the public and the media in the area of food safety we *recommend* that both the DH and MAFF consider arrangements for providing simple but informative briefing to the public and media at appropriate intervals. (3.45)

R.3.7 We *endorse* the DH's intention to consider ways of encouraging more complete notification. We also *recommend* that some guidelines on the case definition of food poisoning should be developed since this would assist uniformity of notifying practices across the country. (3.49)

R.3.7 This will be considered alongside the present review of the notification system for infectious diseases.

R.3.8 We *recommend* that the CDSC and Department of Enteric Pathogens (DEP) databases should be co-ordinated so that this potential source of confusion in the salmonella isolations data is eliminated. (3.46)

R.3.8 The need for this has been recognised by PHLS and the two databases are already being reconciled.

R.3.9 We *recommend* that CDSC with the rest of PHLS take steps to improve the routine central reporting of outbreaks by laboratories and local authorities, particularly the outbreaks occurring in institutions and those affecting the community at large (as opposed to family outbreaks). (3.22)

R.3.9 The Government agrees that central reporting of outbreaks should be encouraged. Although existing arrangements are voluntary the PHLS is looking at ways of improving reporting.

R.3.10 We *recommend* that DH, the Welsh Office and the PHLS Board discuss the organisational arrangements in the context of the management of surveillance of foodborne disease and infectious intestinal disease with a view to improving co-ordination and effective interaction. (3.47)

R.3.10 The Government accepts this recommendation.

R.3.11 We therefore *recommend* that the Steering Group on the Microbiological Safety of Food which we propose in Chapter 5 should consult the Office of Population Censuses and Surveys (OPCS), the PHLS and the SVS with a view to the harmonisation of data collection and reporting wherever this would not result in a loss of useful information. (3.50)

R.3.11 The Government agrees with this objective and will consider how best to achieve it wherever possible.

R.3.12 The Government should use its best efforts to encourage standardisation of data collection and reporting with respect to food-poisoning micro-organisms internationally and throughout the European Community as quickly as possible. (3.51)

R.3.12 The Government will encourage standardisation of data collection where possible.

LOCAL SURVEILLANCE STRUCTURES

Training of Environmental Health Officers (EHOs) and Consultants in Communicable Disease Control (CCDCs)

R.4.1 It is essential that the training of both MO's EH (CCDCs) and EHOs enable them to take effective and coherent action to control food poisoning outbreaks. The establishment of Control of Infection Committees as suggested in 'Public Health in England' is a useful development which we fully support. (4.28)

R.4.1 and 4.2 The Government agrees with the Committee on the importance of appropriate training for CCDCs and notes the Committee's views expressed in their letter.

R.4.2 So important did we feel that the recruitment and training of potential CCDCs should be pursued with vigour that we wrote to the Secretary of State for Health outlining our concerns. A copy of our letter and the Secretary of State's reply are at Annex 4.2. (4.40)

R.4.3 (a) Institutes of Higher Education (including especially the new Schools of Public Health) should be encouraged to mount training programmes for CCDCs. These programmes should also be available for Veterinary Officers and Environmental Health Officers working in this area.

(b) The centres running training courses for EHOs should liaise with the Institution of Environmental Health Officers to ensure the courses have a uniform and adequate content dealing with food safety issues.

(c) The advent of the CCDCs will inevitably involve some changes in procedure. The Institution of Environmental Health Officers should encourage the development of appropriate short updating courses to familiarise qualified EHOs with the changes in the arrangements for public health at local level and the revised arrangements for the notification of communicable disease. (4.43)

R.4.3 (a-c) These recommendations are chiefly for the medical profession, the Institution of Environmental Health Officers and the training bodies. The Government endorses these proposals.

Local surveillance structures — management of outbreaks

R.4.4 We *recommend* the Steering Group on the Microbiological Safety of Food should be asked to consider the matter [introduction of arrangements to aid tracing back] in detail and to make recommendations. (4.32)

R.4.4 The Government agrees that this should be considered although as the Committee points out practical difficulties will have to be taken into account.

R.4.5 There is a need for a code of practice giving guidance on the management of outbreaks. We *recommend* the Steering Group should give early attention to the need to produce this code.

R.4.5 The Government agrees that this should receive early attention.

Review of the Law on Infectious Disease Control

R.4.6 We *recommend* as follows:—

(a) Both local authorities and health authorities should have a specific statutory duty to provide an infectious disease control service.

(b) The statutory responsibility for leading and co-ordinating the services should lie with the health authority, but strong links are needed with local authority EHOs.

(c) The concept of the "proper officer" should be retained: with regard to notification of disease the "proper officer" should be medically qualified.

(d) The statutory notification of disease should go to the "proper officer" who would normally be the CCDC, but this information will also need to be passed on to the relevant environmental health department immediately if it relates to a case of food poisoning.

(e) The CCDC should be the designated person to lead and to co-ordinate the response to an outbreak of food poisoning at local level. The CCDC should also constitute the link between peripheral PHLS and DH centrally, and the local authority and the National Health Service at local level. The prime position of the CCDC should be clearly stated in any Codes of Practices that are produced.

(f) We realise that the move towards the clearer demarcation of responsibilities may throw up difficulties for the CCDC in ensuring the availability of adequate resources within the local authority. Consideration should be given to this potential problem in the development of a Code of Practice for outbreak management.

R.4.6 These recommendations will be taken into account along with comments from other bodies on the proposals in the consultation document published by the Department of Health in October 1989.

(g) A national director of contact points at local authority and health authority level should be developed, if possible, to also include details of the most useful industry links, which can aid in outbreak management. (4.44)

R.4.6 (g) The Government accepts this recommendation and has already set the work in hand to revise the present list of contact points that are appropriate for food hazard management.

NATIONAL SURVEILLANCE STRUCTURES

R.5.1 We see a need for a national microbiological surveillance and assessment system. (5.19) We *recommend* that such a system should be set up. (5.22) There will also be a need for a structure to assess the results of this surveillance in the context of the food chain and epidemiological information on human and animal diseases. (5.23)

R.5.2 We therefore propose a structure which involves two committees:—

(i) A Steering Group to co-ordinate microbiological food safety.

(ii) an Advisory Committee to provide an independent expert view on the public health implications of food safety matters and in particular on the results of the surveillance. It will also advise on the areas where surveillance and other Government activities are needed. (5.32)

R.5.3 We are clearly of the opinion that the lead should be with the Department of Health. (5.41)

R.5.4 Although we recommend a separate committee structure for microbiological food safety to work alongside the existing system for dealing with chemical safety, we nevertheless consider it important that these two groups should not work in total isolation from one another. We *recommend* that steps should be taken to achieve effective communication between the two, and believe some consideration should be given to a degree of cross-membership. In our judgement this applies, in particular, to the two Steering Committees. (5.39)

R.5.1-R.5.4 The Government agrees in principle on the need to strengthen microbiological food surveillance and in particular on the need to co-ordinate activity and to draw on independent expertise. It is considering the detailed arrangements for this.

R.5.5 We *recommend* that this Steering Group should consider with the food industry what information they can make available to central government. (5.9)

R.5.5 The Government accepts this recommendation in principle.

R.5.6 We *recommend* that Local Authorities, the Department of Health and the Welsh Office should encourage Environmental Health Departments wherever possible, to target their surveillance work more precisely in future and to carry out whenever possible, well founded surveys to provide good quality information as a sound basis for decision making. (5.17)

R.5.6 The Government accepts this recommendation.

POULTRY MEAT PRODUCTION, MONITORING AND SURVEILLANCE

R.6.1 We *recommend* the Government should establish a monitoring programme to determine the extent of contamination with pathogenic bacteria at the successive stages of the poultry meat production chain and in the end product of the abattoir operation. In addition to providing baseline information, this should enable a comparison to be made between the bacterial strains in poultry and those found in humans. We would envisage the Steering Group being involved in devising this programme. (6.7)

R.6.1 The Government will consider what monitoring or surveys can most cost effectively be carried out.

R.6.2 Periodic surveys of the incidence of salmonella in broiler flocks are required to establish the effect of MAFF's measures on the incidence of salmonella in broilers (6.33)

There is a need, at each successive stage of broiler production, for more targeted studies to establish the effectiveness of the measures that have been introduced to minimise contamination and to determine whether further measures are needed. We strongly recommend that appropriate studies should be implemented urgently. (6.44)

R.6.2 The Government is fully committed to evaluating its policies and will continue to monitor the effectiveness of the measures in reducing salmonella infection.

R.6.3 We *recommend* that research on the origin of these Campylobacter [in poultry flocks] and the possibilities for control should be undertaken urgently. (6.10)

R.6.3 The Government accepts the desirability of research in this area and will consider further when drawing up research programmes.

185

R.6.4 We *recommend* that MAFF's two data series [from the recently introduced legislation] should be kept under close scrutiny by the proposed Steering Group in order to determine whether further action is required. (6.22)

R.6.4 The Government accepts this recommendation in principle: the data will be examined closely to identify changing patterns.

R.6.5 We *recommend* that the poultry industry should apply the principles of Hazard Analysis Critical Control Points.

R.6.5 This recommendation to the industry is endorsed by the Government whose measures on salmonella are aimed at critical control.

Poultry Meat Production — Feeding Stuffs

R.6.6 We *recommend* to the Government and the industry that urgent consideration should be given to correcting the shortcomings in the feeding stuffs production process. The Steering Group should be involved in this consideration. (6.25)

R.6.6 Codes of Practice for the control of salmonellae have been introduced which include the production of final feed for live stock. Work is almost completed on a survey on contamination of feed ingredients. The need for further measures will be kept under review.

R.6.7 We *recommend* that the Government should keep the microbiological status of vegetable-derived proteins under review, and be ready to introduce regulations if this proves necessary. (6.26)

R.6.7 The survey of feed ingredients referred to above will cover vegetable protein. The results together with reports of salmonella isolations under the Zoonoses Order will provide a basis for considering what further action may need to be taken.

R.6.8 We *recommend* that the Government should keep under review the adequacy of the code of practice on rendering; should closely monitor compliance with the code, and be prepared to translate some of its provisions into law if necessary. We see the Steering Group being involved in this monitoring. (6.21)

R.6.8 The Government accepts this recommendation. The Government has doubled the rate of inspections of rendering plants; these visits provide an opportunity to monitor compliance with the code and to identify problem areas.

R.6.9 We *recommend* that processed animal protein must be effectively separated from the raw material, and must be hygienically handled and stored and transported from the production plant in lorries that have been properly cleansed before use. (6.19)

R.6.9 The Government endorses the recommendation. Advice on this subject is contained in the Code of Practice for the Control of Salmonella in the Animal By-Products Rendering Industry.

Poultry Meat Production — Broilerhouses

R.6.10 Some poultry houses are not up to the appropriate standard because they still have earth floors that cannot effectively be disinfected in between batches. Such unsuitable housing should be phased out wherever possible. We believe close attention also needs to be paid to the supply and distribution of drinking water, which is a likely source of campylobacter infection. One way of controlling the route of infection may be by chlorination of the water supply. We *recommend* that the Government should produce guidelines on the hygienic design of broilerhouses, including their water supply and distribution systems. The Government should also collect appropriate microbiological data in this area. (6.34 and 6.35)

R.6.10 The Government agrees on the need to discourage unsuitable forms of poultry housing although the variety of different systems (including free range) has to be recognised; further consideration will be given to the recommendations on water supplies and the design of broilerhouses. The Government will consider the most appropriate methods of collecting data.

Poultry Meat Production — Distribution and Transport

R.6.11 We *recommend* the Government issue guidance to producers and slaughterers — and where appropriate to the enforcement authorities — on the most desirable practices for transportation to slaughter. (6.37)

R.6.11 The Government agrees. Guidance has already been drawn up and will be issued to the enforcement authorities shortly.

R.6.12 [Improvements in the design of cage systems now permit more effective disinfection than hitherto.] We *recommend* the older design of crate should be phased out as quickly as possible. (6.37)

R.6.12 There is already a move towards the new design of crate, which the Government agrees is to be encouraged. In the meantime, the Government will advise local authorities on the need to ensure that crates are properly cleaned.

R.6.13 We *recommend* that the Government should consider amending the Poultry Meat (Hygiene) Regulations to require the decks of lorries to be cleansed and disinfected, in addition to crates, as soon as practicable after delivery of consignments. (6.37)

R.6.13 The Government agrees on the need for better cleansing of lorries. However, this is subject to European Community legislation and it will be necessary to agree the matter on a Community basis before the regulations can be amended. In the meantime, the Government will incorporate advice into the guidance which is shortly to be issued to local authorities and the industry.

**Poultry Meat Production —
Slaughterhouses**

R.6.14 We *recommend* that ease of cleaning should in future be a high priority for those designing the equipment. (6.39)

R.6.14 The Government agrees on the need for ease of cleaning to be a high priority in the design of equipment. As most equipment used in meat plants is produced and used in Europe, the Government will raise the matter on a European basis.

R.6.15 The evisceration process should be thoroughly re-evaluated, with particular attention being paid to the design of the machinery and whether the viscera should remain attached to the carcase until inspection. (6.39)

R.6.15 The evisceration process is subject to European Community legislation. The Government will raise these points as part of a general review of the inspection system which is already under way.

R.6.16 For reasons of microbiological safety we must *recommend* that scalding [of chicken carcasses] should be carried out at the highest temperature that is practicable. (6.39)

R.6.16 The Government agrees and will discuss this with the industry to establish whether there are ways of overcoming the problems associated with higher scald temperatures.

R.6.17 We *recommend* that giblets should only be sold separately from (and certainly not within) poultry carcasses. (6.39)

R.6.17 The Government will explore this with the industry and in the European Community.

**FOOD MANUFACTURING
PROCESSES**

R.7.1 We *recommend* to the Government, that together with local authorities and the food industry, they should establish food categorisation on this basis [according to microbiological risk]. (7.6)

R.7.1 The Government already distinguishes between foods, processes and premises according to risk; and they will consider whether this approach can be further developed.

R.7.2 The Committee is concerned that some companies may not have sufficient in-house expertise to be able to establish whether a particular process produces a microbiologically safe product. We therefore *recommend* that companies should draw on appropriate expertise, either by joining a suitable Research Association or by having recourse to recognised consultants or other sources of expert advice. (7.18)

R.7.2 The Government endorses the principle that companies should ensure that they have the necessary expertise available.

R.7.3 We welcome the fact that the Government is proposing in the Food Safety Bill to take power to make regulations requiring operators to take expert advice on the safety of particular processes. We further *recommend* that this power should be activated promptly and should include ensuring the safety of the process if changes are made. (7.19)

R.7.3 The Government proposes to take powers under Clause 16 of the Food Safety Bill; the details, after consultation, will be introduced through regulations.

R.7.4 We *recommend* that the Institute of Food Science and Technology (IFST) should take the initiative in reviewing the existing codes, in defining gaps and future needs, and in co-ordinating the production and continued updating of codes of practice. (7.37)

R.7.4 The Government endorses this recommendation and hopes that the IFST will be able to do this.

R.7.5 We *recommend* that all food processing procedures should be designed on Hazard Analysis Critical Control Points principles operated by properly trained staff using validated control programmes in premises with appropriate hygienic facilities. Local authority enforcement officers should seek to encourage this through inspection activities and to ensure that if changes to the process are made the manufacturer checks that this does not adversely affect the microbiological safety of the end product. (7.34)

R.7.5 The Government endorses this recommendation and supports the principle that food industry and enforcement authorities should take systematic account of food safety requirements.

R.7.6 Managers and supervisors must be properly trained as they need to understand the microbiologically important aspects of the processes for which they are responsible. Management should take explicit responsibility for food safety training. (7.28)

R.7.6 This recommendation will be considered in the context of the recent consultation document on training.

R.7.7 We *recommend* that professional staff in environmental health departments should receive appropriate training in food microbiology, food technology and food control systems, including the HACCP system and its applications, sufficient to enable them to know when there is a need to call in more expert sources of advice to assess the more complex processes. (7.38)

R.7.7 The Government endorses this recommendation.

Food Manufacturing Processes — legislative aspects

R.7.8 We *recommend* that the Government should exercise particularly stringent controls over the processes mentioned in Annex 7.2 and 7.3 in order to minimise the risk of food poisoning from these processes. These processes should be considered for licensing under the new powers taken under the Food Safety Bill. (7.40)

R.7.8 The Government accepts the importance of particularly stringent controls for sensitive processes. The Government has announced its intention of introducing tighter controls on food processes which involve vacuum packing. This process covers most of the processes referred to by the Committee. The Government will be issuing draft regulations to control the production, storage and distribution of vacuum packed and other hermetically sealed products. These regulations will tighten the controls on these processes considerably. For pre-cooked chilled meals generally there are existing codes of practice which lay down detailed guidance; and the new Food Hygiene Regulations will require special temperature controls. The Government considers that these arrangements will provide the stringency of control which the Committee identifies as necessary.

R.7.9 We *recommend* that the Government, in reviewing the Food Hygiene Regulations after the passage of the Food Safety Bill, should take into account the importance of construction and design, and should develop central guidelines on the application of these regulations at local level, as suggested in our first letter to Ministers of 24 August 1989 (see Annex 9.1). We welcome the Government's recently declared plans to set up an Implementation Advisory Committee (7.21)

R.7.9 The Government accepts this recommendation.

Food Manufacturing Processes — Design of equipment

R.7.10 The proper design of equipment and correct installation and running of processes is highly important in the control of food contamination and hence in reducing food poisoning risks. We believe it is the responsibility of the food manufacturing industry to ensure that the equipment is suitable for its purpose. We *recommend* that the Food and Drinks Federation should take the lead in promoting a dialogue between food equipment manufacturers and the food industry aimed at improving hygienic design, and at establishing formal arrangements for the approval and certification of food manufacturing equipment. (7.26)

R.7.10 This is a matter for the industry; the Government endorses this recommendation.

FOOD PROCESSING BY SMALL ENTERPRISES

R.8.1 We *recommend* that central government should take the lead in consulting all interested parties and in compiling an information pack for smaller food processing businesses. (8.10)

R.8.1 The Government is sympathetic to this recommendation and will explore with the interested parties how best to take it forward.

R.8.2 There is a complementary need for central guidance to EHOs. (8.11)

R.8.2 The Government agrees with this recommendation which will be taken forward in the context of the Implementation Advisory Committee which it is setting up.

R.8.3 Smaller food processors should in our view be subject to licensing arrangements once the Food Safety Bill is enacted, to the extent that they engage in the kind of sensitive processing operations we have identified in Chapter 7 as worthy of consideration for licensing. (8.12)

R.8.3 This is covered by the response to R.7.8.

THE LEGISLATIVE FRAMEWORK

Licensing and Registration

R.9.1 We feel that, in order adequately to protect the public health, there is considerable advantage in prior inspection and approval before a food business is opened or a process started, whether as part of a "Registration" or a "Licensing" procedure. (9.8)

As we have made clear in our letters to Ministers (Annex 9.1), we believe a system of formal licensing involving prior inspection should in due course be extended to a wide range of food operations including all catering establishments and those premises carrying out butchery and processing of meat. We also believe a similar licensing system should apply to some processes used in the preparation of food (notably the process of manufacturing pre-cooked chilled products, low-acid canning, aseptic packaging of food and vacuum packing including the "sous vide" system) because of the potential dangers that arise when these processes are poorly carried out. (9.9)

R.9.1 The Government is taking a general power in the Food Safety Bill to require food premises to be registered or additionally to operate in accordance with a licence. Registration is intended to help enforcement officers build up a clear picture of the food and catering industry in their area and hence to help set enforcement priorities. It would operate in conjunction with the powers relating to improvement notices, prohibition orders and emergency prohibition notices and orders. The Government intends to require a very simple form of registration of all commercial and permanent food premises and that the intention to open a new business should be lodged with the local authority at least 4 weeks before the business opens, thus enabling the local environmental health department to inspect the premises at an early stage where appropriate. Registration is, however, clearly of right and penalties for failure to register within the due period should not be set at a level which is disproportionate to the offence. When an existing business changes hands, details of the change of ownership should be notified, though not necessarily within the same timescale. Special arrangements will need to be made for those businesses already in existence when the regulations come into force.

Licensing would be used where a category of food business needs to be subject to especially tight control to ensure that they are operated safely. The Government intends to use this power to licence food irradiation facilities, dairy farms and dairies. It proposes to use other powers to control some of the processes mentioned by the Committee (see response to Recommendation 7.8). It also is considering the arrangements needed for regular inspections of food premises under the Official Control of Foodstuffs Directive. It considers however that a wider requirement for licensing would be an unreasonable burden.

R.9.2 We also believe that any licencing procedure adopted should include within it a requirement for the business or process to employ adequately trained personnel. The need to ensure a sufficient supply of such trained personnel is a further reason that the more extended licensing we would recommend will need to be introduced in a carefully co-ordinated fashion. (9.10)

R.9.2 In those particular areas where the Government is contemplating licensing (see R.9.1 above), it will take this recommendation into account in its consultations.

R.9.3 We recognise that such a formal licensing system may take time to implement and we have therefore suggested that, in the first instance, the Regulations, whether for registration or for licensing, should be so worded as to require notification to the enforcement authority of intent to open or operate a business or process 4 to 6 weeks before operations begin. (9.12)

R.9.3 See response to R.9.1.

Moreover such an arrangement [an initial inspection before opening and subsequent inspections at annual intervals] need not in our view require more resources overall than are likely to be needed anyway to implement the [Official Control of Foodstuffs] Directive. (9.14)

R.9.4 One practical and resource-sparing measure which we believe would enable enforcement authorities to achieve a more adequate level of monitoring than they do at present would be to encourage the development of a new cadre of specialist food technicians who would be available to assist EHOs. (9.15)

R.9.4 The Government agrees with the need for EHOs to have specialist food expertise available and looks to the Institution of Environmental Health Officers to pursue this recommendation.

Labelling of Food

R.9.5 We make the following recommendations to Ministers with the aim of ensuring that the potential improvements in microbiological food safety are secured:—

(a) the Government should introduce the compulsory "use by" system as soon as practicable, and phase out the old "sell by" system at the same time so as to avoid a multiplicity of date-marking systems;

R.9.5 (a) The Government has already agreed with the other member states amendments to the European Community labelling rules which will phase out "sell by" dates and introduce "use by" dates for foodstuffs that are microbiologically highly perishable. The relevant changes to the UK Food Labelling Regulations will be proposed shortly.

(b) the Government should issue clear guidance to help ensure that manufacturers and enforcement officers all have a common appreciation of what products are to be regarded as "highly perishable" and thus as subject to the new "use by" requirements;

R.9.5 (b) The Government has already indicated to interested parties that it proposes to discuss with them the criteria that should be used in assessing whether a foodstuff qualifies as "microbiologically highly perishable" and thus has to carry a "use by" date marking rather than the more general "best before" marking.

(c) the Government should also issue guidance to food manufacturers on how to determine shelf life for particular products when deciding on their "use by" date. This guidance might need to stress that shelf lives for individual products can only be determined in the light of proper consideration of the particular product by a suitably qualified microbiologist. It could usefully, however, also set out some general principles. We would expect one of these to be that where a highly perishable product is used as an ingredient in a further product without further processing, the "use by" date cannot be later than that on the original product;

R.9.5 (c) The determination of shelf life for a foodstuff and therefore the allocation of the appropriate date marking can only be done by the food manufacturer or handler who will be aware of composition, manufacturing process and likely storage and handling conditions to which the food has been or will be subject. It follows that if the food manufacturer or handler is to discharge this responsibility effectively, he must as appropriate resort to expert advice. Such advice is already available from a number of sources in both the public and private sectors.

(d) the Government should make it an offence for retailers to sell food for human consumption or for caterers to use it, after its "use by" date;

R.9.5 (d) During the consultation on the draft regulations to introduce "use by" dates, the Government will consult interested parties on whether the sale of foodstuffs once "use by" dates have expired should be illegal.

(e) the Government should remind consumers from time to time of the meaning of the "use by" date and of the risks of not observing it. (9.5)

R.9.5 (e) The Government has already explained the significance of date marking in its booklet "Look at the Label" and has also given advice on the handling and storage of food in the home in its booklet "Food Safety". Both booklets can be obtained free of charge by writing to Food Sense, London SE99 7TT. The Government keeps its publicity in this area under review and when necessary seeks advice on food labelling matters from the Food Advisory Committee.

Refrigerators

R.9.6 We gather that MAFF is seeking to get temperature performance criteria recognised at the Community level. We strongly endorse this position. We firmly believe that — in view of its importance for microbiological food safety — provisions on the ability of refrigerators to hold food at a stated maximum temperature should be given the force of law at the European Community level. We strongly urge that this is brought about at an early date. (9.28)

R.9.6 The Government welcomes the support of the Committee for the line that it is already taking.

APPENDIX 2

BOTULISM

A2.1 This Appendix gives a brief review of foodborne botulism in the UK and refers to some possible implications of the outbreak which took place in North-West England and North Wales in June 1989.

THE ORGANISM

A2.2 *Clostridium botulinum* is a strictly anaerobic, spore-forming bacillus. Seven distinct types designated A to G are now recognised, differentiated by the serological specificity of the toxins which are produced during growth. Taxonomically *C.botulinum* can be divided into two main groups; Group I are mesophiles and grow between about 12°C and 45°C; Group II are psychrophiles and grow between 3.5°C and 48°C. *C.botulinum* spores are widespread in soil and occur in both salt and freshwater mud and in the intestinal tracts of animals, including fish. Variations in the frequency and types isolated from the environment have been reported in countries throughout the world. In the UK non-proteolytic type B strains (Group II) predominated in samples of offshore sediments and mud collected from inland lakes and waterways in the 1970's; types C, D, E, and F were also present but type A was not found[1]. The spores are either moderately or highly heat resistant; thus those of type A and proteolytic types B and F survive boiling for several hours, although those of type E and non-proteolytic types B and F are rapidly destroyed between 95°C and 100°C. In contrast, the toxins of all types of *C.botulinum* are moderately heat-labile and are inactivated by heating at 80°C for 30 minutes[2].

CLINICAL FEATURES

In animals

A2.3 Outbreaks of botulism occur in animals including poultry, due to *C.botulinum* types C and D, but in the UK nearly all reports have been of type C. Human disease due to these types has not been substantiated. In some fish, for example trout, low concentrations of type E spores are common, and type E may cause disease in the fish. Types A and B and non-proteolytic types B and F also may occur in fish from estuarine and coastal waters. Types A and B have sometimes been isolated from cattle, sheep and pigs. These spores may contaminate the fish or meat flesh at slaughter and subsequently lead, through poor handling procedures, to botulism in humans.

In humans

A2.4 *C.botulinum* types A, B and E account for almost all cases of recorded foodborne botulism. "Classical" botulism is due to the consumption of food containing pre-formed toxin. Infection with *C.botulinum* has also been recognised in infants at weaning; "infant botulism" follows the ingestion of spores resulting in colonisation of the gut and the production of toxin and is typically a much milder illness than "classical" botulism[3]. A similar infection with *C.botulinum* has also been suspected in adults in patients with underlying gastrointestinal disease. Botulism has also been reported caused by the organisms growing and producing toxin in wounds.

A2.5 *C.botulinum* toxin is a potent neurotoxin, and the symptoms and signs are predominantly those of muscular paralysis. They usually begin between 18 and 36 hours after the ingestion of the toxin but the incubation period ranges from 6 hours to 8 days. The first symptoms are commonly blurring of vision or double vision due to paralysis of the ocular muscles, followed by difficulty in speaking and in swallowing as the paralysis extends downwards. The mouth and throat become very dry. Vomiting and mild diarrhoea are frequent early symptoms; abdominal distention and pain, and constipation may occur. There is no sensory loss, although paraesthaesiae have been reported in some cases, and the patient remains mentally alert. Fever is absent early in the illness but may develop later, usually due to chest infection when paralysis involves the respiratory muscles. Death is usually due to respiratory failure or inhalation pneumonia. In general, the shorter the time between consuming contaminated food and the onset of symptoms, the more severe the disease and the higher the case fatality rate. Mild and atypical cases occur, and botulism due to type B toxin may be less severe than that due to type A[4]. However, the case fatality rate is usually high, although much less than in the past before the introduction of intensive respiratory care. The most important factors in survival remain the prompt diagnosis, early administration of antitoxin on suspicion of the diagnosis as well as supportive therapy[5].

A2.6 Laboratory confirmation is by the demonstration by mouse protection tests of *C.botulinum* toxin in the patient's serum and/or gastrointestinal tract, and/or in suspected food. Cultures of suspected food, and of the patients faeces and vomit, may give positive results; but the isolation of the organism is, alone, of relatively little significance whereas the detection of toxin provides unequivocal evidence to support the diagnosis. Identification of *C.botulinum* in the laboratory is difficult as its biochemical and fermentative properties are unremarkable; apart from the production of toxin it is indistinguishable from *C.sporogenes*, a saprophyte frequently found in raw food[5].

MODE OF OCCURRENCE

A2.7 *C.botulinum* is ubiquitous and can be isolated occasionally from many different foods, but botulism does not occur unless circumstances permit the growth of the organism and production of toxin in food, which is then eaten cold or without sufficient cooking to inactivate the toxin. These circumstances include an anaerobic environment, a pH not lower than 4.6, adequate available moisture, a low concentration of salt, and sufficient time at a temperature at which the organism will grow (Table A2.1). Such circumstances have occurred most often in preserved foods such as salted, smoked or fermented fish and meat products and in defectively home canned or home bottled low acid foods such as vegetables. The foods implicated differ between countries and are commonly defectively canned or bottled home-produced, low-acid vegetables in the United States, cured or smoked meats in Northern Europe, home preserved vegetables in Italy and Spain and marine products in countries where type E botulism occurs. Indeed, the different patterns of botulism throughout the world are largely a reflection of the eating

Table A2.1 **Minimal requirements for growth and heat resistance of** *C. botulinum* **types A,B,E, and F**

Properties	Group	
	I*	II**
Toxin types	A,B,F	B,E,F
Inhibitory pH	4.6	5.0
Inhibitory NaCl concentration	10%	5%
Minimal water activity	0.93	0.95
Temperature range for growth	10-48°C	3.3-45°C
Decimal reduction time of spores at 100°C	25 min	<0.1 min

* Proteolytic strains viz. digestion of meat or coagulated protein.
** Non-proteolytic strains.
Modified from Reference 2.

habits and procedures used to preserve foods in different societies[6]. In the UK "high risk" foods are not normally eaten and canned and bottled foods are mainly produced commercially, providing some of the microbiologically safest foods available.

A2.8 However, there are new potential hazards associated with changes in food processing and preservation such as extended life cook-chill, sous-vide catering, vacuum packaging, reductions in nitrite levels in cured meats, and the tendency to use lower cooking temperatures than in the past to reduce loss of yield and improve the colour and texture of the products.

A2.9 One hazard of particular importance arises because non-proteolytic Group II strains of *C.botulinum* can grow slowly at refrigeration temperatures (Table A2.1), and mild heat treatments followed by vacuum or modified atmosphere packing may select for these organisms[7] (see Chapter 6 on Fish and Shellfish).

A2.10 Other hazards may arise because of changes in food processing. For example, the outbreak of type B botulism in North West England and North Wales in 1989 was due to yoghurt containing a particular batch of hazelnut conserve. This conserve had been produced without sugar, to reduce its calorie content, and sweetening was provided with aspartame[8]. Without sufficient sugar this low acid product then provided a suitable culture medium for *C.botulinum*. The episode drew attention to the need for manufacturers to obtain expert advice on new or changed food processes before these are introduced (see Part I, paragraph 7.18 and 7.19).

TRENDS IN DATA

A2.11 Foodborne botulism has been reported from many countries and there are marked variations in incidence[2]. There are also variations in the distribution of types, for example, type A predominates in China, the Eastern States of the United States and Argentina, type B in Central Southern Europe and type E in Japan, Canada, Scandinavia and Iran.

A2.12 Botulism is very rare in the UK. In total, ten separate incidents have been reported with 56 cases and 18 deaths (Table A2.2). Four were due to type A toxin, one of which was a single case in a person who acquired the disease abroad, one each to B and E and in three the type was not known. In the first reported outbreak at Loch Maree, Scotland, in 1922, eight people were affected, all of whom died, after eating sandwiches made from bottled wild duck paste. Between this outbreak and the 1989 outbreak, 21 cases with 9 deaths were reported in eight separate incidents. A wide variety of foodstuffs was implicated[9].

Table A2.2 **Foodborne botulism in the UK**

| Year | Number of | | Food vehicle | *C.botulinum* type |
	Cases	Deaths		
1922	8	8	Duck paste	A
1932	2	1	Rabbit & pigeon broth	?
1934	1	0	Jugged hare	?
1935	5?	4?	Vegetarian nut brawn	A
1935	1	1	Minced meat pie	B
1947	5	1	Macaroni cheese	?
1955	2	0	Pickled fish from Mauritius	A
1978	4	2	Canned salmon from USA	E
1987*	1	0	Kosher airline meal	A
1989	27	1	Hazelnut yoghurt	B

*Patient acquired the disease from food prepared abroad.
Modified from Reference 9.

A2.13 The most recent outbreak due to hazelnut yoghurt was caused by type B toxin and comprised 27 cases, including only one death. It was the first incident since 1947 due to UK produced food. On the 8 June 1989 several cases of suspected Guillain-Barré syndrome occured in Preston and Blackpool, but when on the following day two children from the same family were admitted to a hospital in Manchester, a provisional diagnosis of botulism was made. Intensive epidemiological investigation identified hazelnut yoghurt as the likely vehicle of infection. Despite initial negative tests for *C.botulinum* toxin in the sera of two patients, the epidemiological evidence was sufficient to warrant stopping production and withdrawal of the yoghurt on 11 June. This rapid public health response almost certainly prevented a much larger outbreak[8].

A2.14 In this incident there were several mild and atypical cases which together with their widespread geographical distribution and the novel vehicle of infection made diagnosis difficult[10]. It is possible that this may herald a change in the epidemiology of botulism in the UK, similar to that which has taken place in the United States, where larger outbreaks due to newly identified food vehicles have occurred[11] as a consequence of changes in the types of food and in raw materials and their increasingly widespread use. Outbreaks may therefore become more widely spread geographically and in time, new vehicles of infection may occur, and furthermore some cases, particularly of type B botulism, may present with mild and atypical clinical features. These changes in the epidemiology and clinical presentation of botulism, which were apparent in the recent UK outbreak[10], demonstrate the need for improved surveillance systems to facilitate the early detection of widespread outbreaks and the rapid identification of possible food vehicles.

CONCLUSIONS

A2.15 Botulism is a very rare disease in the UK but the 1989 outbreak of 27 cases emphasised the need for continued vigilance in the manufacturer of "high risk" low acid foods and the provision of expert microbiological advice to all manufacturers of these products. Furthermore, such advice is especially important when milder processes requiring less heat and less preservatives are used, or modified atmospheric packaging, including vacuum packaging, is used for extended shelf-life refrigerated foods. Surveillance systems should be developed to detect quickly geographically widespread cases of acute neurological disease which might be due to mild or atypical botulism.

References

1. BALL AP, FARRELL ID. Review. Problems in human botulism. Journal of Infection 1979; **1**: 121-125.

2. HAUSCHILD AHW. *Clostridium botulinum.* In Foodborne Bacterial Pathogens. Doyle MP, ed. New York: Marcel Dekker Inc. 1989. P 111-189.

3. ANONYMOUS. Infant Botulism. Lancet 1986; **2**: 1256-1257.

4. HUGHES JM, BLUMENTHAL JR, MERSON MH, *et al.*Clinical features of types A and B foodborne botulism. Annals of Internal Medicine. 1981; **95**: 442-445.

5. GILBERT RJ, WILLIS AT. Memorandum Botulism. Community Medicine 1981; **2**: 25-27.

6. MEYER KF. The status of botulism as a world health problem. Bulletin of the World Health Organization 1956; **15**: 281-298.

7. CONNER DE, SCOTT VN, BERNARD DT, KAUTTER DA. Potential *Clostridium botulinum* hazards associated with extended shelf-life refrigerated foods: a review. Journal of Food Safety 1989; **10**: 131-153.

8. O'MAHONY M, MITCHELL E, GILBERT RJ, *et al.* An outbreak of foodborne botulism associated with contaminated hazelnut yoghurt. Epidemiology and Infection 1990; **104**: 389-395.

9. GILBERT RJ, RODHOUSE JC, HAUGH CA. Anaerobes and food poisoning. In Clinical and Molecular Aspects of Anaerobes. Boriello SP, ed. Petersfield, England: Wrighton Biomedical Publishing Ltd. 1990. P85-89.

10. CRITCHLEY EMR, HAYES PJ, ISAACS PET. Outbreak of botulism in North West England and Wales, June 1989. Lancet 1989; **2**: 849-853.

11. MACDONALD KL, COHEN ML, BLAKE PA. The changing epidemiology of adult botulism in the United States. American Journal of Epidemiology 1986; **124**: 794-799.

APPENDIX 3

VIRAL FOODBORNE DISEASE

A3.1 This appendix gives an account of foodborne viral gastroenteritis and viral hepatitis in the UK. Both are specifically human infections which do not occur in animals.

THE INFECTIOUS AGENTS A3.2 A viral cause for acute gastroenteritis was first demonstrated in a school outbreak in Norwalk, Ohio, USA, which took place in 1969. The virus was later detected by electron microscopy of stool filtrates, and became known as Norwalk agent[1]. Similar viruses were found in subsequent outbreaks in the USA and elsewhere and because they could not be grown were classified by their size, morphology and buoyant density[2]. Those viruses referred to as small round structured viruses (SRSVS) or Norwalk-like agents are now considered to be the commonest cause of foodborne viral gastroenteritis in the UK[3]; in over 90 per cent. of outbreaks where virus was detected it was a member of this group[4].

A3.3 Hepatitis A virus (HAV) is to date the only reported cause of foodborne viral hepatitis in the UK. In other parts of the world hepatitis E virus, which is also enterically transmitted, is an important cause of severe hepatitis spread by sewage contaminated drinking water[5]. HAV is a small symmetrical RNA virus which has recently been propagated in cell culture and is now classified as enterovirus type 72[6]. In phosphate buffered saline solution the virus is destroyed instantaneously at a temperature above 85°C, but it is probably more heat stable when suspended in protein rich solutions[7]; it is inactivated in cockles by heat treatment giving an internal temperature of the meat of 85-90°C for one minute[8]. HAV resists acid conditions (pH 3), non-ionic detergents, indefinite cold storage at 5°C and prolonged freezing at −20°C. Indeed, refrigeration and freezing are recognised means of preserving viruses in the laboratory. Both HAV and SRSVs are therefore likely to survive for long periods on contaminated refrigerated or frozen foods.

CLINICAL FEATURES A3.4 Viral gastroenteritis caused by SRSVs is reported more frequently in adults than in children. It is a self-limiting disease, usually mild and of 24-48 hours duration, although sometimes symptoms persist for up to two weeks. The incubation period is longer than in acute bacterial foodborne disease and ranges from 15 to 50 hours; it may be dependent on the dose of the infecting virus. Symptoms begin very suddenly and include malaise, nausea, abdominal pain, vomiting, which may be projectile, and diarrhoea. These features togther with a high secondary attack rate due to person-to-person spread are characteristic of SRSV outbreaks[4]. Routine laboratory confirmation depends upon the demonstration of the virus particles in the stools or vomit by electron microscopy, but this is only likely to be successful within 48 hours of the onset of symptoms when the virus is present in sufficient numbers. Other more sensitive laboratory methods are being developed, but are not yet available for routine use; however, recent reports that parts of the genome of the Norwalk agent have been cloned indicate that sensitive and rapid molecular tests are likely to be developed in the near future[9].

A3.5 <u>HAV infection</u> is most common in young children when it is often symptomless or gives rise to a mild illness. Although the infection is much less frequent in adults, the severity of the disease is greater and this increases with age[6]. The mean incubation period is four weeks, when there is usually a gradual onset of anorexia, malaise, pyrexia and vomiting, followed 4 to 10 days later by the development of jaundice. Complete recovery is usual within a few weeks, but in adults, it may be prolonged for several months. Rarely fulminating disease occurs, particularly in older adults. Death may follow[5], most frequently in the elderly[6]. Laboratory confirmation of HAV infection is usually by serological tests for IgM antibody, but tests for the detection of HAV antigen in the stools are also used.

MEANS OF INFECTION

A3.6 The transmission of SRSVs and HAV is similar; both commonly spread directly from person-to-person by the faecal-oral route, but they also spread by the contamination of food and water. The viruses do not grow outside the human body, and food or water serve only as a mechanical carrier. There are not routine tests available for detecting these viruses in food or water; the infecting dose is probably low and a small number of viruses in food cannot usually be detected by electron microscopy because the technique is not sufficiently sensitive.

A3.7 Viral contamination of food may occur at any stage in the food chain, but usually during production or later during preparation or serving[4]. Molluscan shellfish have been the most frequently reported vehicles of viral foodborne disease; they concentrate virus particles during feeding in sewage polluted water and these are not always subsequently removed by current methods of depuration (see Chapter 6). Outbreaks of HAV infection in the UK have been traced to frozen raspberries probably contaminated during picking[10]. The use of human slurry as a fertilizer on strawberries was thought to be the source of a large outbreak in Czechoslovakia.

A3.8 Infected foodhandlers have been implicated as the source of outbreaks due to the contamination of food during preparation; the food vehicles are typically those which are handled in the kitchen and served cold, such as salads, fruit, cake icing, sandwiches and cold meats[1]. Human "carriers" of SRSVs and of HAV have not been conclusively demonstrated. SRSVs are usually excreted shortly before the onset of symptoms, are found in very large numbers in faeces and vomit during the illness, decrease rapidly within 24 hours of recovery and may persist in the stools for at least 48 hours[1]. HAV appears earlier in the stools, up to two weeks before the onset of clinical hepatitis, but excretion then diminishes rapidly and is usually considered to have ceased by seven days after the onset of jaundice; virus excretion takes place for a similar period in persons in whom HAV infection is sub-clinical.

A3.9 The contamination of foods by faecally soiled hands is probably the commonest mode of spread of foodborne viruses in the kitchen, but spread by environmental contamination and from raw foods such as shellfish may also occur. A recent epidemiological study of an hotel outbreak of gastroenteritis due to SRSVs suggested that sudden projectile vomiting contaminated the environment, including working surfaces and stored foods[11]. Furthermore, investigation of outbreaks aboard cruise ships has demonstrated the importance of environmental contamination of cabins and toilet areas by vomit in the spread of SRSVs[12].

TRENDS IN DATA

A3.10 Reported outbreaks of viral foodborne disease increased in the UK during the 1980's. The first confirmed outbreaks of foodborne gastroenteritis due to a virus took place in the South of England in 1976 and 1977 and were associated with the consumption of cockles harvested from sewage polluted waters and which had been inadequately cooked[13]. In 1978 an outbreak of hepatitis A infection in the Midlands and North of England was traced to mussels which had also been harvested from a sewage polluted estuary and inadequately cooked[14]. In a widespread outbreak of hepatitis A infection in 1980 and 1981 mainly affecting the South of England, an epidemiological study demonstrated an association between illness and eating cockles[15].

A3.11 A review of shellfish-associated disease in England and Wales between 1941 and 1983 showed that although bacterial infections declined, those with a viral or suspected viral cause increased, particularly during the 1970s and early 1980s. Part of this increase may have been due to improved surveillance following the introduction of better laboratory methods to identify these infections. The outbreaks were mainly due to inadequately cooked cockles or to raw oysters[16]. More recent data provided by CDSC recorded 95 outbreaks of illness traced to molluscan shellfish between 1981 and 1988, comprising 5 due to HAV, 20 to SRSVs and a further 69 probably caused by SRSVs though not microbiologically confirmed. Only 1 was of bacterial origin.

A3.12 PHLS studies on the inactivation of HAV in cockles by heat treatment[8] led to the design of new heat processing equipment for cockles which was installed in 1988 at Leigh-on-Sea, Essex[4], a major cockle producing area for the South of England. Since this time there have been no reported outbreaks of viral illness from this source, although shellfish which have not been adequately heat treated have continued to be associated with illness. However, the winters of 1988 and 1989 were mild in the UK and outbreaks of viral illness previously have followed very cold weather when heat treatment may have failed[17]. Oysters are usually eaten raw and will continue to pose a hazard to health until effective methods of cleansing and depuration to eliminate viruses are devised.

A3.13 Outbreaks of foodborne viral disease due to foods other than molluscan shellfish were also reported but were less common. Most notable were several outbreaks of HAV infection due to frozen raspberries; these were probably caused by contamination by workers during picking or weighing the raspberries prior to freezing[10]. Five other outbreaks of HAV infection were reported to CDSC during the 1980s all of which were probably due to contamination of food during preparation by infected food handlers. One was caused by iced buns prepared by a school pupil who later developed mild anicteric HAV infection, one by salad prepared by a chef who had serological evidence of recent HAV infection, and one to bread contaminated by a shop keeper with mild HAV infection[18]. In the other two outbreaks a precise link with a food handler was not recorded. Riordan[3] listed 13 outbreaks of foodborne SRSV gastroenteritis not caused by shellfish, in 8 of which there was illness in food handlers and in 3 more of which there was microbiological evidence of infection in foodhandlers; the food vehicles were salads in 4 outbreaks and a variety of mainly cold foods in the remainder. The prevention of spread of viral foodborne disease from infected foodhandlers depends upon the continuous maintenance of high standards of personal and food hygiene (see Chapters 9 and 10) and the exclusion of staff when ill. Present knowledge indicates that exclusion should continue for at least 2 days after recovery from viral gastroenteritis and for 7 days after the onset of jaundice in viral hepatitis.

A3.14 There are limited routine data on SRSVs with which to assess trends; laboratory reports increased during the 1980s which was mainly due to more frequent examination of specimens during outbreaks, and reached a peak of over 350 in 1987 at a time when cockle-associated outbreaks were taking place. More routine data were available for HAV infections, which include statutory notifications of "infective jaundice" (viral hepatitis) since 1969 and laboratory reports since 1980. Notifications in England and Wales fell from over 23,500 in 1969 to just over 3,200 in 1979 and in Scotland by a similar proportion from over 5,200 to under 400 respectively (Table A3.1), which was attributed to a decline in HAV infection[19]. There were subsequently two peaks in both notifications and laboratory reports, one in 1982 and the other in 1989 in England and Wales and at about the same time in Scotland, probably due to long-term natural variations in infection. The apparent paradox of a substantial decline in HAV infection at the same time as a rise in foodborne disease may be explained by a fall in endemic infection spread by the faecal-oral route in children as standards of hygiene and sanitation have improved. This has resulted in more persons reaching adult life without immunity acquired by natural infection, who therefore are likely to succumb to illness when exposed to sewage contaminated shellfish or other faecally contaminated foods containing HAV.

Table A3.1 **Notifications of infective jaundice/viral hepatitis and laboratory reports of hepatitis A virus infection: England and Wales, and Scotland 1969 to 1989**

Year	Notifications		Laboratory reports	
	England and Wales	Scotland	England and Wales	Scotland
1969	23,580	5,218		
1970	21,584	3,801		
1971	14,142	2,634		
1972	12,269	1,765		
1973	8,073	1,121		
1974	7,620	1,175		
1975	5,756	916		
1976	5,963	853		
1977	5,123	624		
1978	4,675	444		
1979	3,216	386		
1980	5,143	352	1,229	
1981	9,841	515	3,161	215
1982	10,605	853	4,928	563
1983	6,316	1,054	2,644	703
1984	5,805	1,077	2,838	620
1985	4,382	907	2,470	297
1986	3,630	514	2,438	202
1987	3,379	511	2,994	368
1988	5,063	848	4,578	642
1989 provisional	7,701	831	5,331	626

Note:
Notifications of "infective jaundice", from 1969 in England and Wales, and "acute infective jaundice" in Scotland. In 1975 in Scotland and in 1988 in England and Wales these were changed to "viral hepatitis".
Source: OPCS, CDSC, CD(S)U.

CONCLUSIONS

A3.15 There was a reported increase in viral foodborne disease in the UK during the 1980s due both to HAV and SRSVs, mainly conveyed by shellfish harvested from sewage polluted waters, but also by foods contaminated during preparation by infected foodhandlers.

A3.16 Improved methods of heat treatment of cockles introduced in 1988 are likely to lead to a decline in cockle-associated disease, but oysters, which are usually eaten raw, will continue to transmit infection until methods of treatment are developed to remove viruses. Infected foodhandlers are an important source of infection and may contaminate the kitchen environment as well as foods; high standards of personal and food hygiene, and exclusion from work of ill staff are necessary to interrupt this mode of transmission.

References

1. ANONYMOUS. Norwalk agent comes of age. Journal of Infection 1990; **20**: 189–192.

2. CAUL EO, APPLETON H. The electron microscopical and physical characteristics of small round human faecal viruses: an interim scheme of classification. Journal of Medical Virology 1982; **9**: 257–265.

3. RIORDAN T. Norwalk virus disease. In: Morgan-Capner P, ed. Current topics in virology. London: PHLS 1991. In press.

4. APPLETON H, CAUL EO, CLEWLEY JP, *et al.* Foodborne viral gastroenteritis. PHLS Microbiology Digest 1988; **5**: 69–75.

5. ZUCKERMAN AJ. Hepatitis E virus. British Medical Journal 1990; **300**: 1475–1476.

6. FORBES A, WILLIAMS R. Changing epidemiology and clinical aspects of hepatitis A. British Medical Bulletin 1990; **46**: 303–318.

7. PARRY JV, MORTIMER PP. The heat sensitivity of hepatitis A virus determined by a simple tissue culture method. Journal of Medical Virology 1984; **14**: 277–283.

8. MILLARD J, APPLETON H, PARRY JV. Studies on heat inactivation of hepatitis A virus with special reference to shellfish. Epidemiology and Infection 1987; **98**: 397–414.

9. ESTES MK, GRAHAM DY, WANG K, JIANG X. Molecular characterisation of the genome of Norwalk virus. Gastroenterology 1990; **98**: A447.

10. REID TMS, ROBINSON HG. Frozen raspberries and hepatitis A. Epidemiology and Infection 1987; **98**: 109–112.

11. REID JA, CAUL EO, WHITE DG, PALMER SR. Role of infected food handler in hotel outbreak of Norwalk-like viral gastroenteritis: implications for control. Lancet 1988; **2**: 321–323.

12. HO MS, GLASS RI, MONROE SS, *et al.* Viral gastroenteritis aboard a cruiseship. Lancet 1989; **2**: 961–956.

13. APPLETON H, PEREIRA MS. A possible virus aetiology in outbreaks of food-poisoning from cockles. Lancet 1977; **1**: 780–781.

14. BOSTOCK AD, MEPHAM P, PHILLIPS S, *et al.* Hepatitis A infection associated with the consumption of mussels. Journal of Infection 1979; **1**: 111–177.

15. O'MAHONY MC, GOOCH CD, SMYTH DA, *et al.* Epidemic hepatitis A from cockles. Lancet 1983; **1**: 518–520.

16. SOCKETT PN, WEST PA, JACOB M. Shellfish and public health. PHLS Microbiology Digest 1985; **2**: 29–35.

17. APPLETON H. Foodborne viruses. Lancet 1990; in press.

18. WARBURTON ARE, WREGHITT TG, RAMPLING A, *et al.* Hepatitis A outbreak involving bread. Epidemiology and Infection 1990; in press.

19. PHLS Communicable Diseases Surveillance Centre and the Communicable Diseases (Scotland) Unit. Communicable Disease Report. Community Medicine 1985; **7**: 211–216.

APPENDIX 4

OTHER RELEVANT PATHOGENS

A4.1 There have been major changes in the pattern of foodborne infectious disease in the UK in the past few decades[1]. Typhoid and paratyphoid fevers have declined from around 1,000 cases per year in the early 1940s to less than 300 in the 1980s, about 85 per cent. of them in persons who acquired the infection abroad, and foodborne spread in the UK is now rarely reported. Although over 50 cases of cholera due to the El Tor biotype have been imported since 1970, further transmission of the disease in the UK has not followed. The major milkborne zoonoses, tuberculosis due to *Mycobacterium bovis* and brucellosis, have been controlled (see Chapter 5 Milk and Milk Products). Foodborne tapeworm infestations due to *Taenia solium* and *T.saginata* are now rarely reported and are usually acquired abroad, and fascioliasis and trichinosis have been virtually eliminated as indigenous diseases. At the same time other foodborne diseases have increased, notably salmonellosis, and several pathogens, either previously unrecognised or hitherto not known to be foodborne, have emerged. Two of the most important of these were described in Part I of the Report, namely *Campylobacter* and *Listeria monocytogenes*. This Appendix briefly describes some other pathogens relevant to the UK which may cause foodborne illness. Verocytotoxin producing *Escherichia coli*, *Yersinia enterocolitica*, *Aeromonas hydrophila*, and *Vibrio parahaemolyticus*, all of which are infections, *Clostridium perfringens*, *Staphylococcus aureus*, *Bacillus cereus* and other *Bacillus* spp, the toxins of which cause food poisoning, and two protozoa, *Giardia lamblia* and *Cryptosporidium*.

VEROCYTOTOXIN PRODUCING *ESCHERICHIA COLI*

A4.2 Pathogenic strains of *E. coli* have been described as belonging to three main groups; enteropathogenic strains (EPEC) classically associated with infantile gastroenteritis, enterotoxigenic strains (ETEC) particularly associated with "travellers diarrhoea", and enteroinvasive strains (EIEC) causing a dysentery-like illness[2]. All three groups can be transmitted by food or water but are not important causes of foodborne or waterborne disease in the UK. A fourth group is now recognised in which the strains produce cytotoxins which affect Vero (African green monkey kidney) cells. This group, known as Verocytotoxin producing *E. coli* (VTEC), are a cause of foodborne illness with a wide range of disease from mild diarrhoea to the life threatening conditions, haemorrhagic colitis, thrombotic thrombocytopaenic purpura and the haemolytic uraemic syndrome (HUS)[3].

The infectious agent

A4.3 VTEC is a gramnegative non-sporing bacterium. It grows over a similar temperature range to salmonellas, 10°C to 50°C, and grows optimally at about 37°C. The organisms survive refrigeration but are readily killed by pasteurisation and by chemicals such as chlorine. Verocytotoxin (VT) is now known to comprise at least two distinct types of toxin designated VT1 and VT2, both of which appear to be involved in the pathogenesis of human disease; the biological activity of VT1 is similar to the toxin produced by *Shigella dysenteriae* type 1, and has also been described as shiga-like toxin (SLT1)[3]. Many different serogroups of *E. coli* produce VT, but 0157 has been that most frequently isolated from humans[3]; however, this may be partly due to selective routine laboratory screening for these sorbitol-negative strains with MacConkey-sorbitol agar[4]. A phage-typing scheme for VTEC 0157 has been developed in Canada and recently applied in the UK, which is likely to provide valuable epidemiological information for the detection and investigation of outbreaks[5].

Clinical features

A4.4 In animals in the UK, MAFF routine data show that VTEC has been isolated from cattle and pigs and has been associated with enteric disease in young animals and oedema disease in pigs, but VTEC 0157 has not been found. In a study of 24 bovine and 14 porcine strains of VTEC[6], 20 bovine strains produced VT1 or VT2 but not both, and all of the 14 porcine strains produced VT2 only. The bovine strains comprised 9 different O serogroups and the porcine 6, but none of them were 0157. Three of the porcine strains were isolated from cases of oedema disease. In only one UK study, in an abattoir in Sheffield, was serotype 0157 isolated from cattle, where 2 of 207 faeces samples were positive[7].

A4.5 In humans VTEC is a cause of haemorrhagic colitis which is characterised by severe abdominal pain, bloody diarrhoea and little or no fever. It affects people of a wide age range but mainly adults. There is usually full recovery, although occasionally deaths have been reported, principally in the elderly[4]. In outbreaks the disease has an incubation period of between 3 and 8 days with a maximum of about 12 days[8]. It has a seasonal peak in the summer months. HUS comprises acute renal failure, thrombocytopaenia and haemolytic anaemia; it is more common in children than in adults and is the commonest cause of acute renal failure in children in Western Europe and North America[9]. In adults a similar condition, thrombotic thrombocytopaenic purpura, also occurs associated with VTEC. Two types of HUS are recognised in children, one of which is preceded by diarrhoea, 'typical HUS' or 'D+ HUS' and in the the UK appears to be usually due to VTEC and shows the same summer seasonal peak in incidence as haemorrhagic colitis. It is less severe than 'atypical HUS' or 'D− HUS', which is not associated with VTEC, but nevertheless can cause death and permanent renal damage. In a review of 70 cases of 'typical HUS' seen in London between 1980 and 1986, there was a case fatality ratio of 6% and of those who recovered about 13% had some degree of renal impairment[10].

Mode of transmission

A4.6 Foodborne infection due to the consumption of undercooked food products of animal origin, usually bovine, appears to be the commonest mode of transmission in North America, but direct person-to-person transmission may also occur[3]. In England in two outbreaks a possible vehicle of infection was suggested; in one, the handling of fresh vegetables was associated with disease[8], and in the other cold turkey roll was implicated epidemiologically[11], but in neither was the source of infection found. In only the one study, in Sheffield, was bovine infection suggested as a possible source[7]. Thus, in the UK the main sources and modes of transmission of VTEC are not known but epidemiological evidence suggests that the infection may be foodborne.

Trends in data

A4.7 Before the early 1980s VTEC 0157 infection appears to have been rare in the UK; a study of 15,000 isolates stored by the PHLS Division of Enteric Pathogens showed that only 2 were serogroup 0157[12]. However, an outbreak of HUS associated with diarrhoea in North Wales in 1963[13] suggested an infective agent as the cause, and it is possible therefore that strains of VTEC could have been present in the population at that time. Nevertheless, the now frequent isolation of VTEC, particularly serogroup 0157, probably indicates a real increase in incidence, although some of the increase may be due to greater clinical detection of haemorrhagic colitis and HUS and the more frequent laboratory examination of specimens. Isolations of VTEC 0157 are now reported routinely. In 1989 there were 118 reports in England and Wales and 86 in Scotland; proportionately a much higher rate in Scotland than in England and Wales, possibly due to an active surveillance system, with increased interest of microbiologists, which began in Scotland in January 1989.

A4.8 Although routine data are not available on trends in haemorrhagic colitis a study in 1985/86 showed evidence of VTEC infection in 39% of 89 cases, two of which were fatal; 30 of 32 strains were serogroup 0157[4]. A passive surveillance scheme for HUS in the British Isles began in 1983 and in the first two years 77 cases were reported[14]. Although there was under-reporting, the introduction of active surveillance by the British Paediatric Surveillance Unit in 1986, and a special study with the PHLS Division of Enteric Pathogens between 1985 and 1988[9], suggested that there may have been a real increase in incidence. Data from the British Paediatric Surveillance Unit showed that in the UK in 1989 there were 188 reported cases (181 D+ HUS including 5 deaths) compared with between 83 and 130 per year in the years 1985-88. In the 1985-88 study there was evidence of VTEC infection in 58 of 185 (31%) samples, in 38 of which the VTEC strains isolated were serogroup 0157[15]. In an earlier study by the PHLS Division of Enteric Pathogens of 66 patients between 1983 and 1985, 22 (33%) had evidence of VTEC infection and 15 of 19 VTEC strains examined were serogroup 0157[16]. However, the proportion of cases associated with VTEC may be much higher than around one-third because isolation rates of the organism are greater earlier in the disease; in the 1985-88 study over 60% of samples collected in the first three days of the prodomal illness were positive[9]. Recent studies by the PHLS Division of Enteric Pathogens indicate that an even higher proportion of cases of HUS may be associated with VTEC; up to 80% may show evidence of infection, mainly with serogroup 0157. This laboratory also showed that in haemorrhagic colitis many other VTEC serogroups occur.

YERSINIA ENTEROCOLITICA

A4.9 *Y.enterocolitica* was first described in 1939 as a human pathogen, and received its present name in 1964 because of its association with intestinal infection[17]. Reported infections increased substantially in many parts of the world, particularly in cooler climatic areas during the 1970s and 1980s and outbreaks of foodborne disease were described[17].

The infectious agent

A4.10 *Y.enterocolitica* is a gram negative non-sporing rod shaped bacterium. It grows over a wide temperature range 0°C to 40°C, similar to *Listeria monocytogenes*, with optimum growth at about 29°C. It is motile at 25°C and non-motile at 37°C. It can be classified into biotypes, serotypes and phage types and by plasmid analysis[17]; biochemical marker tests for presumptive virulence using calcium deficient culture medium have been used to distinguish pathogenic from non-pathogenic strains[18]. Serotypes 03 and 09 are those most commonly reported in humans in Europe and 08 in the United States, although 03 has recently been recognised more frequently in that country[19]. Laboratory diagnosis is by isolation of the organism, which usually takes one to two weeks, or by serological methods; cross reactions may occur, particularly between serotype 09 and *Brucella* spp[20], *Y. enterocolitica* is ubiquitous, is widespread in the intestinal tracts of animals and in the environment, including soil and water; pigs appear to be a reservoir of serotypes 03 and 09 in Europe, both of which have been found most frequently in the tongue and tonsils, and also in the caecum. The organism has been isolated from many foodstuffs including meat, particularly pork, dairy products and vegetables[20]. Recent studies by the Public Health Laboratory, Poole, confirmed these findings and reported contamination in over half of 25 samples of salads and coleslaws, but the significance to human disease has yet to be established.

Clinical features

A4.11 The serotypes of *Y.enterocolitica* commonly associated with disease in humans (03, 08 and 09) are not pathogenic to animals but other serotypes have caused illness in chinchillas and hares. The infection itself is of no direct economic importance in farm animals in the UK. However, symptomless infection with *Y.enterocolitica* 09 could present problems in the control of brucellosis, because such infection would give false positive serological reactions. In humans infection most commonly presents after an incubation period of 1 to 11 days as a self-limiting enterocolitis, which lasts between 5 and 14 days but which may persist for several months[17]. The illness is characterised by diarrhoea, abdominal pain which may mimic appendicitis, less frequently vomiting, and fever, accompanied by leucocytosis. It is more common in children than in adults. In children the organisms may persist in the stools for between 2 weeks and 3 months. The infection may be followed by erythema nodosum and arthritis, particularly in adults. Severe complications may occur and are most often seen in persons with underlying disease, and may comprise septicaemia with metastatic abscess formation and other septic infections with a high case fatality rate[17].

Mode of transmission

A4.12 The most frequently documented mode of transmission has been by foods, milk, milk drinks and water[17]. A case-control study in Belgium implicated the consumption of raw pork[21]. Cross-contamination in the kitchen from raw pork chitterlings to prepared infant foods appeared to be the mode of spread to infants in a recent outbreak in the United States[19]. Faecal-oral spread by handling infected pigs, dogs and cats has been reported. Serotypes 03 and 09 may also spread from person-to-person by the faecal-oral route, and this transmission from asymptomatic "carriers" could be a possible explanation of some sporadic cases. Serotype 08 appears to be different; there is no evidence of person-to-person spread and the origin of this serotype is probably more likely to be contaminated water or food[22]. Infection caused by contamination of food by human excreters of the organism has not been described. Transmission by blood transfusion has been reported[17].

Trends in data

A4.13 Laboratory reports of infections due to *Y.enterocolitica* increased in England and Wales from 45 in 1980 to a provisional number of 591 in 1989; reports also increased in Scotland (Table A4.1). Most were sporadic cases, but there were two small school outbreaks, one of which may have been foodborne, and two cases and one symptomless infection, associated with post-pasteurisation contaminated milk, reported to CDSC. Some of the recorded increase is likely to be due to improved methods of detection and better reporting but most of it probably represents a real increase because reports of *Y.pseudotuberculosis* detected by the same methods showed a much smaller increase. Laboratory confirmation of infection is difficult and takes longer than for most other gastrointestinal pathogens so that the reported cases probably underestimate the true incidence of the disease. A study of faecal samples of patients in London[23] and another in Poole[24] gave isolation rates of *Yersinia* spp of 6.1% and 3.5% respectively, but the organisms isolated did not include the serotypes of *Y.enterocolitica* usually recognised as pathogenic to humans in the UK. These studies do not imply, therefore, a substantial under-diagnosis of yersinosis and the incidence of disease in the UK would appear to be much lower than in some other countries such as Belgium, the Netherlands, Canada and Australia[17].

AEROMONAS HYDROPHILA

A4.14 *A.hydrophila* and related species *A.caviae* and *A.sobria* are, like *Y.enterocolitica,* cold tolerant organisms which have also been implicated as a cause of diarrhoeal disease which may be foodborne.

The Infectious agent

A4.15 The *A.hydrophila* group are non-sporing gram negative bacilli which are motile at 25°C but not at 37°C; they grow over a wide temperature range of about 0°C to 40°C with an optimum of 28°C[25]. A serogrouping scheme has recently been extended by PHLS Division of Enteric Pathogens[26]. The organisms are widespread in the aquatic environment, in fish and in other cold blooded animals, and have been isolated from cattle and pigs, from drinking water and many human foods including meat, poultry and raw milk[25]. A recent survey in the Reading area in England demonstrated the organism on raw meat, poultry, offal, fish, cooked meats and pre-prepared salads on retail sale[27].

Table A4.1 **Other relevant pathogens**
Laboratory reports: England and Wales, and Scotland, 1980-89
Number of reports, number of outbreaks in parentheses: 1989 data provisional

Year	Y.enterocolitica		Aeromonas spp		V.para-haemolyticus*	Cl.perfringens		S.aureus		Bacillus. spp		Cryptosporidium		Giardia lamblia	
	E&W	Scot	E&W	Scot	E&W	E&W	Scot	E&W	Scot	E&W	Scot	E&W	Scot	E&W	Scot
1980	45	N/A	71	2	9	1,056(55)	171 (7)	189(11)	2(1)	71(13)	5(1)	N/A	N/A	3,693	237
1981	79	N/A	96	2	9	918(46)	364(10)	143(10)	8(1)	72 (9)	6(1)	N/A	N/A	3,602	225
1982	88	N/A	84	1	14	1,455(69)	95 (6)	89 (7)	14(1)	41(14)	4(1)	N/A	N/A	4,083	224
1983	207	30	174	1	14	1,624(68)	185 (5)	160(14)	25(1)	134(17)	9(3)	61	N/A	4,613	226
1984	237	21	210	—	16	1,716(68)	164 (8)	181 (7)	27(3)	214(24)	—	876	50	5,056	299
1985	409	26	285	26	19	1,466(64)	84 (5)	118(12)	56(3)	81(15)	29(2)	1,874	265	5,095	257
1986	431	67	402	9	11	896(51)	108 (6)	76 (9)	2(1)	65(18)	8(1)	3,560	414	5,680	319
1987	441	46	589	43	18	1,266(51)	149 (5)	178(12)	5(1)	137(21)	12(3)	3,277	493	5,212	305
1988	473	28	467	65	13	1,312(57)	234(11)	111 (9)	5(1)	418(20)	27(5)	2,750	545	5,454	343
1989	591	47	399	79	17	901(54)	75 (5)	104 (8)	18(1)	164(27)	81(4)	7,769	1,243	6,273	357

N/A = not available
*No reports in Scotland

Clinical features	A4.16 In animals, the *A.hydrophila* group may cause disease in fish. In humans, severe extra-intestinal infections including septicaemia have been reported occasionally, usually in patients with underlying malignant or other disease. Cutaneous and pulmonary infections have been reported following swimming or diving accidents. An association with mild self-limiting diarrhoeal disease has been recorded in many parts of the world, particularly in children, and it has been described as a possible cause of "travellers diarrhoea". However, studies in healthy volunteers have so far failed to confirm the intestinal pathogenicity of the organisms[25].
Mode of transmission	A4.17 Direct infection of skin and wounds by contact with contaminated water and pulmonary infection by inhalation of contaminated water occur. Direct or indirect faecal-oral spread from person-to-person has not been demonstrated; foodborne and waterborne infection, although suspected in many incidents, have not yet been fully substantiated[25].
Trends in data	A4.18 In England and Wales and Scotland routine laboratory reported infections with *Aeromonas* spp increased from less than 100 in 1980 to nearly 500 in 1989 (Table A4.1). It is not known to what extent this was a real increase in incidence or a rise due to improved laboratory methods and better reporting. The suspected sources of infection were not recorded in these routine reports.
VIBRIO PARAHAEMOLYTICUS	A4.19 This organism is a frequent cause of food poisoning in warm climates where fish and shellfish consumption is common, but it is a rare and usually imported infection in the UK. A4.20 It is a gramnegative curved rod-shaped organism commonly found in aquatic saline environments at temperatures over 10°C, particularly in coastal and estuarine waters. Illness is usually due to the consumption of raw or undercooked fish or shellfish, or to foods cross contaminated by fish, shellfish or estuarine water. Diarrhoea and abdominal pain follow about 12 hours after consumption of the contaminated food, occasionally with nausea, vomiting and fever. Recovery is usually complete within a few days[28]. A4.21 The disease was first recorded in England and Wales in 1972 and during the 1980s between 9 and 19 cases were reported each year (Table A4.1); there were no cases reported in Scotland. Most cases were infected abroad, some were due to imported cooked peeled prawns and there was one outbreak recorded due to locally caught crab on the South Coast of England[29].
CLOSTRIDIUM PERFRINGENS	A4.22 Although *C. perfringens* was first described as a cause of food poisoning at the end of the 19th Century, it was not until the 1940s that it was shown to be an important cause in the United Kingdom[29].
The organism	A4.23 *C. perfringens* is a grampositive spore forming anaerobic bacillus; the spores are heat resistant and survive cooking; when the vegetative organisms form spores (sporulation) enterotoxin is produced which causes the clinical illness. The optimal temperature for growth is between 43° and 47°C; it will not grow below 10°C. Type A, responsible for food poisoning in the UK, is divided into several serotypes[30]. Laboratory diagnosis is by the demonstration of large numbers of the organisms in the stools of affected persons and in the suspected food, serological confirmation that the strains from both sources are the same, and the detection of enterotoxin in the stools[31]. The spores of the organism are widely distributed in the environment, in soil, in the faeces of animals and humans, and are commonly found in many foods particularly meat, poultry and their products.

| Clinical features | A4.24 Abdominal pain and diarrhoea follow between 8 and 24 hours after eating food containing large numbers of vegetative organisms. Nausea is common but vomiting is unusual. Fever is normally absent. The illness is usually self-limiting and recovery rapid within 12 to 24 hours, although very rarely deaths have been reported in elderly debilitated people. |

Mode of occurrence

A4.25 Although the organism is often present in foods, illness occurs only when there is inadequate temperature control after cooking. The spores survive normal cooking temperatures and times and if a food containing the organisms is then cooled very slowly or is stored at room temperature for a long period, for example overnight, or is reheated slowly, vegetative cells proceed to multiply. When large numbers of organisms are ingested some will be protected in the food from the action of gastric acid and will pass on into the gut to sporulate and produce enterotoxin, giving rise to illness. Meats and meat products are most often involved, especially when these provide anaerobic conditions, such as in stews, pies and gravy.

Trends in data

A4.26 *C. perfringens* food poisoning is a common cause of reported bacterial food poisoning in the UK, although the incidence is much less than that due to salmonellas. Between 1980 and 1989 in England and Wales there were 46 to 69 outbreaks per year, comprising between 896 and 1,624 cases; in Scotland there were between 5 and 11 outbreaks and 75 to 364 cases per year (Table A4.1). Most incidents were reported in closed communities, such as hospitals and homes for the elderly, or in association with meals served in restaurants, hotels or at receptions. Unlike salmonellosis, *C. perfringens* food poisoning did not increase during the 1980s. It is notable that outbreaks reported in hospitals fell from a peak of over 20 per year in the mid-1970s to an average of about half this number during the 1980s. This decline has been attributed to improvements in food hygiene, particularly in methods of temperature control. However, outbreaks in old peoples homes and other institutions remain common and may possibly be increasing.

STAPHYLOCOCCUS AUREUS

A4.27 Toxic food poisoning due to *S. aureus* was described at the end of the 19th century but it was not until the 1930s that its significance as an important cause of food poisoning was appreciated[32].

The organism

A4.28 *S. aureus* is a grampositive coccus, some strains of which produce heat-resistant enterotoxins during growth. There are five main enterotoxins, designated A to E, of which enterotoxin A is most often implicated in outbreaks of food poisoning; the optimum temperature for production of toxin is between 35°C and 40°C[29]. The source of the organism is usually of human origin; it is estimated that about 15 per cent of people in the UK are naso-pharyngeal carriers of enterotoxigenic strains of *S. aureus*, and people with septic lesions or abrasions of the skin are frequently a source of them[29]. Occasionally cattle with staphylococcal mastitis have been implicated as the source of the organism[33]. Laboratory diagnosis is by culture of enterotoxin producing strains of *S. aureus* from the affected persons and/or food handlers and the detection of enterotoxin and/or the culture of the organism from the suspected foods. Phage typing can then confirm that the isolates are all probably the same strain.

Clinical features

A4.29 Nausea, vomiting and abdominal pain, often accompanied by diarrhoea, begin abruptly between 1 and 6 hours after eating food containing enterotoxin. In severe cases there may be dehydration, marked pallor and collapse, which may require treatment by intravenous infusion. The duration of the incubation period and severity of the illness depend upon the amount of enterotoxin ingested. Complete recovery is usual and rapid, within 24 hours, but on very rare occasions deaths have been reported.

Mode of occurrence

A4.30 *S. aureus* is often present on the skin of humans and is probably frequently transferred to food, especially if personal hygiene is poor or if infected skin lesions are not properly protected. However, food poisoning only occurs if a food providing a suitable culture medium is contaminated with enterotoxin producing strains, and is then kept at a suitable temperature for long enough for growth of the organism to produce sufficient enterotoxin. This usually requires a moist food kept for at least 6 hours at room temperature. Cold meats and poultry products are common vehicles of infection, particularly salted meats, because *S. aureus* grows in the presence of concentrations of salt which inhibit the growth of competing microorganisms. Cold sweets such as trifles and cream confectionary are also frequently implicated. Outbreaks due to canned and to bottled products have been reported in the past, probably due to contamination by handling whilst the cans or bottles were cooling and entry of the organisms through minute defects in the seams of the cans or seats of the bottle caps[29].

Trends in data

A4.31 Outbreaks of staphylococcal food poisoning in the UK reached a peak of around 150 per year in 1950s, but declined during the 1960s to between 10 and 20 per year in the 1970s. There were between 7 and 14 reported outbreaks each year with 76 to 189 cases in England and Wales during the 1980s and 1 to 3 outbreaks with 2 to 25 cases in Scotland with no obvious trends (Table A4.1). Few sporadic cases were detected and most of the outbreaks reported were associated with restaurants, hotels, shops or private functions.

***BACILLUS CEREUS* AND OTHER *BACILLUS* SPP**

A4.32 *B. cereus*, although suspected as a cause of food poisoning since the early 1900s, was only established as a generally recognised foodborne pathogen in the 1950s[34]. *B. subtilis* and the closely related species, *B. licheniformis* and *B. pumilus*, have also been associated with outbreaks of foodborne illness in recent years and are now recognised amongst the less common causes of acute bacterial food poisoning in the UK and other parts of the world[34].

The organisms

A4.33 The members of the genus *Bacillus* are grampositive, aerobic or facultatively anaerobic sporing, rod shaped organisms. The mesophilic species which include *B. cereus*, *B. subtilis*, *B. licheniformis* and *B. pumilus*, can grow over a temperature range of 5°C to 55°C with an optimum growth between 28°C and 45°C, depending on the species. The spores are heat resistant and can survive at normal cooking temperatures. The vegetative forms are readily killed by pasteurisation (63-65°C for 28-30 minutes). The organisms are widespread in the environment, in soil, natural waters, vegetation and in many foods, notably cereals and other dried foods, milk and dairy products, meat products and vegetables[34].

Clinical features

A4.34 In animals, *B. cereus* can cause mastitis and abortion in cattle and *B. licheniformis* has been reported associated with bovine toxaemia. In humans, foodborne *B. cereus* gives rise to two types of clinical illness, the "diarrhoeal syndrome" and the "emetic syndrome", caused by different toxins both produced during sporulation of the organism. The "diarrhoeal syndrome" with an incubation period of 8 to 16 hours, comprises watery diarrhoea, sometimes nausea, but rarely vomiting; it is usually associated with proteinaceous foods. The "emetic syndrome" has a shorter incubation period of one to 5 hours, comprises nausea and vomiting, and is sometimes followed by diarrhoea; it is associated with farinaceous foods, particularly cooked rice dishes. *B. subtilis* food poisoning is characterised by acute vomiting after a short incubation period (median 2.5 hours) and *B. licheniformis* by diarrhoea after a longer period (median 8.0 hours); *B. pumulis* food poisoning has an intermediate and variable clinical picture. Recovery from these illnesses is complete and usually occurs within 24 hours[35]. Laboratory diagnosis is by the isolation of the organism from the vomit or faeces of affected persons and the demonstration of large number ($>10^5$/g) of the same organism in the suspected food. Serotyping of *B. cereus* causes non-gastrointestinal infections, particularly of wounds, but also a wide range of more serious conditions such as bacteraemia, septicaemia, ophthalmitis and abscesses, often in immunodeficient or otherwise debilitated people. Similar systemic infections have been occasionally reported due to *B. subtilis* and *B. licheniformis*[35].

Mode of occurrence

A4.35 *B. cereus* spores are frequently present in small numbers in a wide range of foods but food poisoning only occurs following defective food storage after cooking. The spores may survive cooking and if the food is then kept at ambient temperature, spore germination occurs with rapid growth of the vegetative organism to produce a toxic dose. In the UK, where the "emetic syndrome" is commoner than the diarrhoeal syndrome, *B. cereus* food poisoning is usually due to reheated rice dishes[35]. *B.subtilis* and *B. licheniformis* are also present in many foods in small numbers and are an important cause of food spoilage. Again, they only cause food poisoning if circumstances allow their rapid growth to very large numbers. The foods most often implicated are meat pasties, pies and rolls, meat and vegetable stews, bread, crumpets and various oriental meat and seafood dishes[35].

Trends in data

A4.36 Food poisoning due to *B. cereus* and to other *Bacillus* spp was first recorded in the UK in the early 1970s and during that decade there were around 18 outbreaks and 90 cases reported each year. During the 1980s outbreaks increased in England and Wales and in Scotland to 31 in 1989 and the number of cases increased to nearly 250 (Table A4.1). Most of the reported outbreaks were due to *B. cereus* and were associated with fried rice dishes served in ethnic restaurants. More detailed data recorded by the PHLS Food Hygiene Laboratory between 1974 and 1989 showed that during this period 70 outbreaks were due to *B. subtilis* and 32 to *B. licheniformis*, but that these did not increase in the 1980s.

GIARDIA LAMBLIA* AND *CRYPTOSPRORIDIUM

A4.37 These are both protozoa causing gastrointestinal infections which have been recently recognised as important causes of acute diarrhoeal illnesses in the UK.

The infectious agents

A4.38 Both parasites are widespread in animals; *Cryptosporidium* is particularly associated with calves and lambs; *Giardia* appears to be common in domestic dogs and cats in the UK[36] and in North America it has been frequently found in beavers and muskrats. The cysts of both organisms occur in the environment and persist for long periods in water and under moist conditions; those of *Giardia* are oval shaped and between 9 and 12 microns long whereas those of *Cryptosporidium* are about half this size, 4 to 6 microns in diameter. Both are resistant to normal levels of chlorine in water supplies but are killed by boiling[37,38].

Clinical features

A4.39 The clinical features of both diseases are similar and range from mild diarrhoea to profuse watery diarrhoea with foul-smelling stools. However, the incubation period of cryptosporidiosis, 2 to 14 days, is shorter than that of giardiasis, 1 to 4 weeks. The illnesses are self-limiting in healthy people but symptoms may persist for several weeks or even months and particularly in giardiasis may give rise to malabsorption and weight loss. In immunocompromised patients, especially those with AIDS, cryptosporidiosis may cause prolonged and life-threatening diarrhoea. Both illnesses affect all age groups but in the UK cryptosporidiosis is reported most frequently in young children aged 0-4 years and giardiasis in persons aged 15-40 years.

Mode of transmission

A4.40 Giardiasis can be waterborne; spread directly from person-to-person by the faecal-oral route and sexual transmission occurs, particularly in homosexual men; foodborne disease appears to be very rare. Cryptosporidiosis is commonly spread directly from person-to-person, particularly in young children; direct spread from farm animals has often been reported; waterborne spread is also common; there are anecdotal reports of foodborne spread by raw milk and raw sausage meat[38]. Both infections are well recognised infections in travellers ("travellers' diarrhoea"), particularly giardiasis, and occasionally occur together in the same individual. The main area of concern in these diseases is the spread by drinking water because the cysts are resistent to chlorine and may not be entirely removed by filtration, particularly the small cysts of *Cryptosporidium*[37]. In neither infection has foodborne disease yet been confirmed in the UK, but the absence of laboratory tests to detect these protozoa in food severely handicaps investigation[38].

Trends in data

A4.41 Laboratory reports of both *Giardia* and *Cryptosporidium* have increased (Table A4.1). In 1989 in England and Wales there was a provisional total of 6,273 reports of *Giardia* and 7,769 of *Cryptosporidium* and in Scotland 357 and 1,243 respectively. However, a recent PHLS study showed that cryptosporidiosis is more common than these data indicate[39]. Protozoal gastointestinal infections may be more frequently unrecognised that bacterial and viral infections and under-reporting also occurs[38]. It is difficult to determine, therefore, if the recent rises in laboratory reports are due entirely to better recognition and reporting as new laboratory tests have been developed or if they also represent a real rise in incidence.

CONCLUSIONS

A4.42 Campylobacter is the most frequently reported bacterial cause of human gastrointestinal infection to have emerged in the last two decades. Most infections are sporadic and poultry are thought to be the main source. *L. monocytogenes* causes serious disease, continues to be rare and has recently declined; the evidence for foodborne transmission remains unclear (see Part I, Appendices 2 and 3). Infections with Verocytotoxin producing strains of *E. coli* causing haemorrhagic colitis and haemolytic uraemic syndrome have been increasingly recognised, may be rising in incidence and can be foodborne. Although not yet fully assessed, the infection may prove to be an important "new" foodborne disease in the UK. Yersiniosis is probably increasing in incidence and, although there is little evidence so far in the UK to implicate food, it may become a common foodborne disease as in some other countries.

A4.43 Food poisoning due to *C. perfringens*, *S. aureus*, *B. cereus* and other *Bacillus* spp gave rise to between 77 and 110 reported outbreaks per year with from 1,155 to 2,302 cases in England and Wales, and Scotland, during the 1980s, but there is probably considerable under-reporting. Although this group of diseases does not appear to be increasing, they are due to defects in food and/or personal hygiene, principally inadequate temperature control, and are therefore eminently preventable.

A4.44 *V.parahaemolyticus* remains a rare imported foodborne infection, the association of *Aeromonas* spp infections with food remains unconfirmed and although *Giardia* and *Cryptosporidium* are important waterborne infections in the UK, foodborne transmission has not so far been substantiated. None of these pathogens currently pose important problems in foodborne disease in the UK.

References

1. GALBRAITH NS, BARRETT NJ, SOCKETT PN. The changing pattern of foodborne disease in England and Wales. Public Health 1987; **101**: 319-328.

2. GROSS RJ. *Escherichia coli* diarrhoea. Journal of Infection 1983; **7**: 177-192.

3. KARMALI MA. Infection by Verocytotoxin-producing *Escherichia coli*. Clinical Microbiology Reviews 1989; **2**: 15-38.

4. SMITH HR, ROWE B, GROSS RJ, *et al*. Haemorrhagic colitis and Verocytotoxin-producing *Escherichia coli* in England and Wales. Lancet 1987; **1**: 1062-1065.

5. FROST JA, SMITH HR, WILLSHAW GA, *et al*. Phage-typing of Verocytotoxin (VT) producing *Escherichia coli* 0157 isolated in the United Kingdom. Epidemiology and Infection 1989; **103**: 73-81.

6. SMITH HR, SCOTLAND SM, WILLSHAW GA, *et al*. Vero cytotoxin production and presence of VT genes in *Escherichia coli* strains of animal origin. Journal of General Microbiology 1988; **134**: 829-834.

7. CHAPMAN PA, WRIGHT DJ, NORMAN P. Verotoxin-producing *Escherichia coli* infections in Sheffield: cattle as a possible source. Epidemiology and Infection 1989; **102**: 439-445.

8. MORGAN GM, NEWMAN C, PALMER SR, *et al*. First recognised community outbreak of haemorrhagic colitis due to verotoxin-producing *Escherichia coli* 0157.H7 in the UK. Epidemiology and Infection 1988; **101**: 83-91.

9. MILFORD DV, TAYLOR CM, GUTTRIDGE B, *et al*. Haemolytic uraemic syndromes in the British Isles 1985-8: association with Verocytotoxin producing *Escherichia coli*. Part 1: clinical and epidemiological aspects. Archives of Disease in Childhood 1990; **65**: 716-721.

10. LEVIN M, WALTERS MDS, BARRATT TM. Haemolytic uremic syndrome. In: Arnoff SC, ed. Pediatric Infectious Diseases. Chicago: Year Book Medical Publishers Inc. 1989; **4**: 51-81.

11. SALMON RL, FARRELL ID, HUTCHISON JGP, *et al*. A christening party outbreak of haemorrhagic colitis and haemolytic uraemic syndrome associated with *Escherichia coli* 0157.H7. Epidemiology and Infection 1989; **103**: 249-254.

12. DAY NP, SCOTLAND SM, CHEASTY T, ROWE B. *Escherichia coli* 0157:H7 associated with human infection in the United Kingdom. Lancet 1983; **1**: 825.

13. MCLEAN MM, JONES CH, SUTHERLAND DA. Haemolytic-uraemic syndrome. Archives of Disease in Childhood 1966; **41**: 76-81.

14. COMMUNICABLE DISEASE SURVEILLANCE CENTRE. British Paediatric Association — Communicable Disease Surveillance Centre surveillance of haemolytic uraemic syndrome 1983-4. British Medical Journal 1986; **292**: 115-117.

15. KLEANTHOUS H, SMITH MR, SCOTLAND SM, *et al*. Haemolytic uraemic syndromes in the British Isles, 1985-8: associated with Verocytotoxin producing *Escherichia coli*. Part 2: microbiological aspects. Archives of Disease in Childhood 1990; **65**: 722-727.

16. SCOTLAND SM, ROWE B, SMITH MR, *et al*. Verocytotoxin producing strains of *Escherichia coli* from children with haemolytic uraemic syndrome and their detection by specific DNA probes. Journal of Medical Microbiology 1988; **25**: 237-243.

17. COVER TL, ABER RC. *Yersinia enterocolitica*. New England Journal of Medicine 1989; **321**: 16-24.

18 MAIR NS, FOX E. Yersiniosis. London, Public Health Laboratory Service. 1986.

19. LEE LA, GERBER AR, LONSWAY DR, *et al*. *Yersinia enterocolitica* 0:3 infections in infants and children, associated with the household preparation of chitterlings. New England Journal of Medicine 1990; **322**: 984-987.

20. WORLD HEALTH ORGANIZATION. Yersiniosis. Euro Reports and Studies 60. Copenhagen, WHO. 1983.

21. TAUXE RV, VANDEPITTE J, WAUTERS G, *et al*. *Yersinia enterocolitica* infections and pork: the missing link. Lancet 1987; **1**: 1129-1132.

22. CARNIEL E, MOLLARET HH. Yersiniosis. Comparative Immunology, Microbiology and Infectious Diseases 1990; **13**: 51-58.

23. LEWIS AM, CHATTOPADHYAY B. Faecal carriage of *Yersinia* species. Journal of Hygiene (Camb.) 1986; **97**: 281-287.

24. GREENWOOD M, HOOPER WL. Human carriage of *Yersinia* spp. Journal of Medical Microbiology 1987; **23**: 345-348.

25. ALTWEGG M, GEISS HK. Aeromonas as a human pathogen. CRC Critical Reviews in Microbiology 1989; **16**: 253-286.

26. CHEASTY T, GROSS RJ, THOMAS LV, ROWE B. Serogrouping of the *Aeromonas hydrophila* group. Journal of Diarrhoeal Diseases Research 1988; **6**: 95-98.

27. FRICKER CR, TOMPSETT S. *Aeromonas* spp. in foods: a significant cause of food poisoning? International Journal of Food Microbiology 1989; **9**: 17-23.

28. WEST PA. Human pathogenic vibrios — a public health update with environmental perspectives. Epidemiology and Infection 1989; **103**: 1-34.

29. GILBERT RJ, ROBERTS D. Foodborne gastroenteritis. In: Topley and Wilson's Principles of Bacteriology, Virology and Immunity. 8th edition. Volume 3, Chapter 78. Parker MT, Deurden BI, eds, 1990. London: Edward Arnold 1990. P489-512.

30. STRINGER MF, TURNBULL PCB, GILBERT RJ. Application of serological typing to the investigation of outbreaks of *Clostridium perfringens* food poisoning. 1970-1978. Journal of Hygiene (Camb.) 1980; **84**: 443-456.

31. WILLIS AT, PHILLIPS KD. Anaerobic infections. London: Public Health Laboratory Service 1988. P52-54.

32. DACK GM. Food Poisoning. Cambridge: Cambridge University Press. 1956. P109.

33. GALBRAITH NS, FORBES P, CLIFFORD C. Communicable disease associated with milk and dairy products in England and Wales 1951-80. British Medical Journal 1982; **284**: 1761-1765.

34. KRAMER JM, GILBERT RJ. *Bacillus cereus* and other *Bacillus* species. In: Doyle MP, ed. Foodborne Bacterial Pathogens. 1989. New York: Marcel Dekker Inc. P22-69.

35. TURNBULL PCB, KRAMER J, MELLING J. Bacillus. In Topley and Wilson's Principles of Bacteriology, Virology and Immunity. 8th edition. Volume 2, Chapter 9. Parker MT, Duerden BI, eds, London: Edward Arnold 1990. P187-210.

36. WINSLAND JKD, NIMMO S, BUTCHER PD, FARTHING MJG. Prevalence of *Giardia* in dogs and cats in the United Kingdom: survey of an Essex veterinary clinic. Transactions of the Royal Society of Tropical Medicine and Hygiene 1989; **83**: 791-792.

37. REPORT OF A GROUP OF EXPERTS. Cryptosporidium in water supplies. Department of the Environment, Department of Health. London: HMSO. 1990.

38. CASEMORE DP. Foodborne protozoal infection. Lancet 1990; in press.

39. PUBLIC HEALTH LABORATORY SERVICE STUDY GROUP. Cryptosporidiosis in England and Wales: prevalence and clinical and epidemiological features. British Medical Journal 1990; **300**: 774-777.

GLOSSARY

This glossary is included as a general aid to the reader and is not intended to be definitive.

AETIOLOGY

The study of the causation of disease.

ANAEROBE

An organism which can grow in the absence or near absence of oxygen.

ANTHRAX

An acute infective disease, communicable from animals to man. A notifiable disease in animals.

BACILLUS SPECIES

Gram positive aerobic sporing rod-shaped bacteria.

BACTERAEMIA

The presence of bacteria in the blood.

BACTERIUM

A microscopic organism with a rigid cell wall; often unicellular which multiplies by splitting into two.

BRUCELLA

A Gram negative non-sporing bacterium.

CAMPYLOBACTER

A curved Gram negative non-sporing bacterium.

CLOSTRIDIUM BOTULINUM

A Gram positive spore forming anaerobic rod-shaped bacterium.

COLIFORMS

Bacteria whose presence can indicate poor hygiene.

COLONISATION

The phenomenon of a population of microorganisms becoming established in a certain environment (especially in the intestinal tract of humans or animals) without necessarily giving rise to clinical disease.

COMMUNICABLE DISEASE

A disease, the causative organisms of which are capable of being passed from a person, animal or the environment to a susceptible individual.

CONTAMINATION

The presence of pathogenic microorganisms in food, water, in other materials or in the environment or on the body surface of man or animal.

COOK-CHILL

A food production system based on cooking, rapid cooling and chilled storage.

CULTURE (noun)

A liquid or solid medium on or within which has grown a population of particular type(s) of microorganisms as a result of inoculation and incubation of the medium.

CULTURE (verb)

To encourage the growth of particular type(s) of microorganisms under controlled conditions. The resulting population can be used for study and characterisation.

DEMERSAL

Found in deep water or on the sea bottom.

EC DIRECTIVE

Legislation from the European Community that has to be incorporated into member country laws but which leaves to the individual member state to decide how best this should be done.

EC REGULATION

Legislation from the European Community that has to be incorporated directly into member country laws.

EMULSFICATION

Production of a mixture of two immiscible liquids, one being dispersed in the other in the form of fine droplets.

ENTERITIS

Inflammation of the intestine.

ENTEROTOXIGENIC

Able to produce a toxin adversely affecting the intestines.

ENCEPHALITIS

Inflammation of the brain often due to infection with a viral agent.

EPIDEMIOLOGY

The study of factors affecting health and disease in populations and the application of this study to the control and prevention of disease.

EPIDEMIOLOGICAL SURVEILLANCE

The continual watchfulness over the distribution and trends in incidence of disease in a population through the systematic collection, consolidation and evaluation of morbidity and mortality reports and other relevant data. It includes dissemination of information to all those who need to know so that appropriate action can be taken.

ESCHERICHIA COLI

A Gram negative non-sporing rod-shaped bacterium. Found in the gut of man and animals.

EVISCERATION

Removal of the internal organs, including the intestines.

EXSANGUINATION

Removal of the blood.

FEED COMPOUNDING

The manufacture of finished animal diets from a variety of raw materials.

FLOW DIVERSION VALVE

Part of milk pasteurisation plant which prevents inadequately heat treated milk contaminating correctly pasteurised milk.

FOODBORNE ILLNESS

Illness resulting from the consumption of food contaminated by pathogenic microorganisms and/or their toxins.

FOOD HYGIENE

All measures necessary to ensure the safety, soundness and wholesomeness of food at all stages from its growth, production or manufacture until its final consumption.

FOOD POISONING

A notifiable illness normally charcterised by acute diarrhoea and/or vomiting caused by consumption of food contaminated with pathogenic microorganisms and/or their toxins.

FOOT AND MOUTH DISEASE

A contagious disease of cloven-footed animals.

GASTROINTESTINAL INFECTION

Infection of the stomach and intestine usually resulting in diarrhoea and vomiting. This may be due to colonisation of the intestinal tract by pathogenic organisms.

HEAT-LABILE

Unstable at high temperatures.

INDICATOR ORGANISM

Generally a non-pathogenic organism, not normally present in the food, whose presence suggests poor hygiene and that the food could have been contaminated with pathogenic organisms.

ISOLATE

A single species of a microorganism originating from a particular sample or environment growing in pure culture.

LABORATORY REPORTS

Data routinely collected nationally of laboratory identifications of certain pathogenic organisms. Includes all those known to cause foodborne infections.

LISTERIA

A Gram positive non-sporing bacterium.

MASTITIS

Inflammation of the mammary gland.

MICROORGANISM

Any organism such as a bacterium or virus.

MORPHOLOGY

The study of the structure and form of microorganisms.

PARTURITION

The act of giving birth.

PASTEURISATION

A form of heat treatment that kills certain vegetative bacteria and/or spoilage organisms in milk and other foods. Temperatures below 100°C are used.

PATHOGEN

Any biological agent that can cause disease.

pH

An index used as a measure of acidity.

PLATE COUNT

Count of the number of colonies of bacteria growing on an agar plate to determine the microbiological status of the sample.

RESAZURIN TEST

Rapid test used as an indicator of microbiological quality of milk.

SALMONELLA

A Gram negative non-sporing rod-shaped bacterium.

SAPROPHYTE

An organism which lives on dead organic matter.

SEROTYPE

A distinct variety within a bacterial species defined by its *in vitro* antigenic reaction.

SPOILAGE ORGANISM

A microorganism causing changes in the appearance, taste or smell of food that are generally regarded to be organoleptically unacceptable.

SPORADIC CASE

A single case of disease apparently unrelated to other cases.

STAPHYLOCOCCUS

A Gram positive coccoid bacterium.

STERILISATION

A process that will kill microorganisms (including bacterial spores). Commercial sterilisation is the destruction of those microorganisms which are able to develop in a particular product under normal storage conditions. A commonly used standard for commercial sterility is the probability of survival of *Clostridium botulinum* spores of 1 in 10.

STREPTOCOCCUS

A Gram positive coccoid bacterium.

THERMODURIC COUNT

Count of organisms which can survive high temperatures.

TOTAL VIABLE COUNT

The number of all those bacteria capable of growth, on the media, in a sample to give a measure of the level of bacteria present.

TOXOPLASMOSIS

A common cause of ovine abortion. The infective agent can cause disease in humans.

TUBERCULOSIS

Infection due to the tubercle bacillus which can be spread by air droplets and raw milk.

VIBRIO PARAHAEMOLYTICUS

A curved Gram negative non-sporing bacterium.

VIRUS

A sub-microscopic non-cellular infective agent that is not capable of self-replication by itself but can reproduce and multiply only in living cells.

WATER ACTIVITY

A measure of the available water in a substance.

YERSINIA

A Gram negative non-sporing rod-shaped bacterium.

ZOONOSES

Diseases which can be transmitted naturally from animal to man and vice versa.

LIST OF ABBREVIATIONS
COMMONLY USED IN THIS REPORT

AFRC

Agricultural and Food Research Council

AMDEA

Association of Manufacturers of Domestic Electrical Appliances

AMI

Authorised Meat Inspector

ASG

Advisory Sectoral Group

ATP

Accord Relatif aux Transports

CCDC

Consultant in Communicable Disease Control

CCP

Critical Control Point

CDSC

Communicable Disease Surveillance Centre (of PHLS)

CD(S)U

Communicable Diseases (Scotland) Unit

CMO

Chief Medical Officer

CPC

Certificate of Professional Competence

CPHM

Consultant in Public Health Medicine

CPHL

Central Public Health Laboratory (of PHLS)

CSA

Common Services Agency (of NHS in Scotland)

CTN

Confectioners/Tobacconists/Newsagents

CVO
Chief Veterinary Officer

DAFS
Department of Agriculture and Fisheries for Scotland

DANI
Department of Agriculture for Northern Ireland

DEH
Department of Environmental Health

DEP
Department of Enteric Pathogens (of CPHL)

DES
Department of Education and Science

DG III
Directorate General III of the European Commission

DG VI
Directorate General VI of the European Commission

DH
Department of Health

DHSS(NI)
Department of Health and Social Security (Northern Ireland)

DVO
Divisional Veterinary Officer

EC
European Community

EHO
Environmental Health Officer

GP
General Practitioner

HACCP
Hazard Analysis Critical Control Point

HMSO
Her Majesty's Stationery Office

IAC
Implementation Advisory Committee

ICMSF
International Commission on Microbiological Specification for Foodstuffs

IEC
International Electrotechnical Commission

IEHO
Institution of Environmental Health Officers

ISD
Information & Statistics Division (of Common Services Agency of NHS in Scotland)

LACOTS
Local Authority Coordinating Body on Trading Standards

MAFF
Ministry of Agriculture Fisheries and Food

MMB
Milk Marketing Board

MRC
Medical Research Council

NHS
National Health Service

NSC
National Surveillance Coordinator

OPCS
Office of Population Censuses and Surveys

OVS
Official Veterinary Surgeon

PHLS
Public Health Laboratory Service

RCDLG
Regional Communicable Disease Liaison Group (in Northern Ireland)

RCGP
Royal College of General Practitioners

RIB
Regional Information Branch (of DHSS(NI))

SAC
Scottish Agricultural College

SFCC
Scottish Food Coordinating Committee

SHHD
Scottish Home & Health Department

SI
Statutory Instrument

SRSV
Small Round Structured Virus

SVS
State Veterinary Service (of MAFF)

TBC
Total Bacterial count

UK
United Kingdom

VFS
Veterinary Field Service

VIC
Veterinary Investigation Centre

VIDA
Veterinary Investigation Diagnostic Analysis

VIS
Veterinary Investigation Service (of SVS)

WHO
World Health Organization

Printed in the United Kingdom for HMSO   Dd293579   1/1991